BOOK

WITHDRAWN

The Hospice Handbook

A COMPLETE GUIDE

LARRY BERESFORD

Foreword by Elisabeth Kubler-Ross

LITTLE, BROWN AND COMPANY

Boston   Toronto   London

First Edition

Library of Congress Cataloging-in-Publication Data

Beresford, Larry.
    The hospice handbook: a complete guide / by Larry Beresford.
       p.   cm.
    Includes bibliographical references.
    ISBN 0-316-09138-3
    1. Hospice care—Handbooks, manuals, etc.   I. Title.
R726.8.B36   1993
362.1'75—dc20   92-32814

10 9 8 7 6 5 4 3 2 1

RRD-VA

Published simultaneously in Canada by Little, Brown & Company (Canada) Limited

Printed in the United States of America

*To my hospice volunteer coordinators, and to the
wonderful folks at Coming Home Hospice;*

*and to my mother, Barbara Gale Beresford, who
knew where she was going and said her
good-byes before she left, and my father and stepmother,
Bruce Comstock and Joyce Dexter Beresford,
hospice volunteers in Topeka, Kansas*

You matter because of who you are. You matter to the last moment of your life, and we will do all we can not only to help you die peacefully, but also to live until you die.

DAME CICELY SAUNDERS
founder of the
modern hospice movement

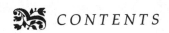 CONTENTS

          and Access Issues   76
          Models of Hospice Programs   76
          Coverage for Hospice Care   84
          Questions Consumers Can Ask a Hospice   96
          Barriers to Hospice Access   101
          Beverly   106

SEVEN   **Pain and Physical Realities**   109
          Betty C.   116

EIGHT   **Legal Issues**   119
          Anna Walton   123

NINE   **The Place for Hope in Hospice**   125

TEN   **Issues in the Future of Hospice**   131
          High Tech and Hospice   133
          Hospice Care for People with AIDS   135
          Children and Hospice   143

          *Afterword: What Does Choosing
          Hospice Really Mean?*   147

          Appendix   151
          *Notes on the Text and Suggestions for
          Further Reading*   157

FOREWORD

Larry Beresford's *Hospice Handbook* is a thorough study of the evolution of America's hospices in the last twenty years. I feel honored to be able to add a few words to this tremendous undertaking, with the hope of encouraging more people to investigate hospices in their neighborhood and to discuss the issues with their next of kin so that if there is ever a need for such terminal care within the family, people know their options and have already done their "shopping around" before they are in crisis.

If I look back thirty years (as of this writing in 1992), I see that the United States has made tremendous strides in terminal care and that patients now finally have an option and something to say about the whereabouts and the place of their final care. Thirty years ago, practically all patients died in a hospital setting, an institution, or a nursing home without much choice about the quality and the quantity of their final care. It was a big, traumatic event, usually, when somebody was diagnosed to be terminally ill, with the expectation of horrendous pain, very inadequate pain management, and very little open discussion about the terminal illness. Ten years later (twenty years ago), things had changed tremendously; a great percentage of patients were choosing to die at home with a prepared family member taking most of the burden and the care and a few visiting nurses dropping in and helping by moving or turning the patient or maybe giving a bath. With the occurrence of the newly modified Brompton's mixture, which was a great step forward for pain relief in the early seventies, we started planning, discussing, hoping, and preparing for the building of a hospice in Connecticut. It was a "forceps delivery" and thanks to people like Florence and Henry Wald and other friends with great foresight and tenacity, after four years the ground was laid in Connecticut for the building of the first hospice in the United States.

Fears were expressed that real estate prices would go down and that nobody would want to live near a "death house." Those fears, naturally, never materialized, and a few years later many, many cities competed to have hospices in their vicinity. It became a competitive struggle over who would have the honor of taking care of terminally ill patients.

The quality of these hospices was very great, as the selection of volunteers was meticulous, with the emphasis on the staff having completed their own unfinished business and not shying away from talking about any issues that the patient would want to discuss. Most of these early hospices were based on voluntary contributions, and there was no political, financial, or government involvement. It was truly in the spirit of the hospice to care for one's fellow man. It is only in the last few years that the requirements started to occur about accreditation, about basic rules and about having not only home care available but also inpatient care for those who could not be taken care of at home. A few years ensued when I questioned the quality of the spirit of the hospices, especially in the early eighties, when the AIDS epidemic made us aware of the need to be much more prepared for what was often a premature and often an unexpected death among the young adults and young-middle-aged people who, due to the AIDS diagnosis, were often rejected, isolated, and treated like leprosy patients. A new fight resulted to ensure that hospices would not discriminate and would take AIDS patients. There were again a handful of hospices that did a marvelous job and became flexible in their rules for admission and treatment and opened their doors wide for their brothers and sisters.

Now, with eighteen hundred hospices in the United States, patients have a choice to spend the last few weeks of their life either in a hospital with all of the technology and life-prolonging procedures or in a hospice. They can choose to die at home with an adequate support system and with visiting nurses, social workers, clergy, and doctors making house calls or can choose a palliative care unit where the emphasis is on comfort care rather than on the prolongation of life.

With MSC, the oral morphine medication, we are now able to take care of the patient's pain in almost 98 percent of cases. The request for active euthanasia has dwindled down to practically zero. If the patient's needs (physical, emotional, intellectual, and spiritual) are taken care of, no patient asks to be "put out of this life." With adequate counseling and the emphasis on the enhancement of the spiritual quadrant, the patients grow in leaps and bounds, and many of my terminal patients have emphasized to me that the last six months of their life were the most valuable months of their entire existence.

Taking care of terminally ill patients is a privilege and a gift which teaches us not only about dying but about living. All of those who have the courage to care for dying patients, either grown-ups or children, black or white, poor or rich, will be enriched by this experience and will contribute to the society, which will ultimately be judged and evaluated by the care of children and terminally ill patients as a reflection of humanity and of true and genuine compassion.

Anyone who has anything to do with hospices or who plans to start a hospice (hospices are especially needed in rural communities), should read this book and will be encouraged to be a catalyst in this world that needs love, compassion, and understanding more than security, money, and material things.

Congratulations to the author and to all of those who contributed to this book to make hospice a viable alternative for the nineties and the future generations of our children and our children's children.

ELISABETH KUBLER-ROSS

ACKNOWLEDGMENTS

I gratefully acknowledge the tremendous encouragement and support that I received from hospice pioneer Zachary Morfogen, for believing in this book and my ability to write it long before I did; from Roger Donald, my editor at Little, Brown, for recognizing its potential and guiding me through the process of clarifying and sharpening its focus; and from Jordan Pavlin, his assistant, for her personal commitment to this project and for her kind words and understanding during the difficult days of rewriting. David Kaplan, author of *Yakuza* and *Fires of the Dragon*, freely offered his invaluable insights and advice on navigating the publishing process. John Mahoney and the staff of the National Hospice Organization have been my best source of information about the American hospice movement, as well as advocates for the highest quality hospice care. My many friends and colleagues among the current and former staff and volunteers of Visiting Nurses and Hospice of San Francisco — far too many of them to list here — have cheerfully answered my countless questions about hospice over the past twelve years. They also provided me with precious training in hospice care and with inspiring models of the practice and the spirit of hospice.

I'd also like to thank Gretchen Brown, Hospice of the Bluegrass in Lexington, Kentucky, and Mary Michal, Hospice-Care of Madison, Wisconsin, for their personal interest and support, and for going above and beyond the call of duty in hosting, organizing, and scheduling my research trips to their states. I'm also grateful, for the hospitality and the valuable information I received at the eight hospices I visited for this book, to Gretchen; Mary; Elaine Cox, Lourdes Hospice in Paducah; Randall DuFour, Hospice of Louisville; Julie Henahan, Hospice of Central Kentucky in Elizabethtown; Norman McRae, Hospice of Hope in Maysville, Kentucky; Sister Rita Adlkofer, St. Joseph's Hospital Hospice Program in Marshfield; James Ewens, Milwaukee Hospice Home Care, both in Wisconsin; and to their agencies' staffs, volunteers, clients, and community physicians who spoke to me.

Michael Rothenberg stepped forward with his poet's eye to review the manuscript at a critical moment. I also received valuable input, advice, and encouragement on all or part of the manuscript from Gail Bigelow, Stephen Connor, James Ewens, Nancy Martin, Mary Michal, True Ryndes, Virginia Shubert, Claire Tehan, Michael Tscheu, Tery Walsh, and my writing group. Many thanks also to everyone I absentmindedly neglected to mention by name.

INTRODUCTION

My first encounter with the hospice concept of humane care for the dying was in 1978, during my final year of studies at the University of Minnesota. I answered a job posting at the student employment service for a part-time secretarial position with the Minnesota Coalition for Terminal Care, a small organization with a one-room office in the University YMCA. I was intrigued by the organization's name and curious to find out why anyone would choose to specialize in issues such as terminal care, death, and dying. The coalition director, Howard Bell, and his assistant, Peter Thoreen, were then busy providing education, coordination, and support to the embryonic hospice community in the Twin Cities and to others involved in the larger field growing up around death and dying issues — death educators, doctors, professors of medical, health, and mortuary sciences, psychologists, and grief counselors.

A week after I started this job, my sister Nancy Martin's husband, David, died in a freak boating accident. She and I would soon spend a lot of time talking about what had happened and what it meant to her. Two months after that my mother was diagnosed with kidney cancer. Following four months of cancer treatment, including surgery, chemotherapy, and several hospital transfers by ambulance, my mother died in a hospital room crowded with my father and most of her seven children and their spouses. Hospice care had not been offered to us. None of her medical professionals suggested bringing her home to die or encouraged a frank discussion of her prospects with the family. One of her doctors had said publicly that he didn't believe in giving patients "death sentences." But she eventually came to know she was dying, anyway, and she was able to say that simple, devastating fact out loud. She talked about her impending death, and her weariness from fighting the disease, with a gentle candor, grace, and even good humor. She found ways to say meaningful good-byes to those she loved, including me.

Those were the first two deaths to have a big impact on my life, the first to involve people who were close to me and yet not elderly, and they shattered the composure of my family. My job at the Coalition suddenly got very interesting. As I typed and filed and answered the phone, I asked questions of Howard and Peter, browsed through the resource library, and tried to learn everything I could about the Coalition's work and the issues it addressed.

A year after my mother's death I moved to California with a journalism degree and a small free-lance writing business. I looked into volunteer opportunities and discovered Hospice of San Francisco, then open just six months, providing care for the terminally ill in their homes. Enlisted by the hospice's volunteer director, Doris Fine, as an office and telephone volunteer on Friday afternoons, I was soon hired by the executive director Stephen Connor as a part-time secretary. Eventually I became office manager.

While I was observing and participating in the administration of this specialized service, I also got involved directly in hospice care as a volunteer working with dying patients. Later I spent four hours a week volunteering at Coming Home Hospice, the model fifteen-bed residential hospice facility opened in 1987 by the San Francisco hospice, now called Visiting Nurses and Hospice of San Francisco. Since hospice is care for the dying, and since San Francisco has the country's highest incidence of AIDS (acquired immune deficiency syndrome), it was only natural that VNHSF and volunteers like me soon were also working with people with AIDS. (Today 84 percent of hospice patients nationally have cancer, 4 percent have AIDS, and the rest have a variety of other end-stage illnesses.)

Along the way I began to see how I could put my college journalism training together with my interest in and knowledge about hospice, and I have worked full-time since 1986 as a free-lance writer and editor specializing in hospice management, AIDS care, and related topics for hospice newsletters and other health industry trade publications. That work has provided the foundation for this book.

However, the primary research was done during a trip to Kentucky and Wisconsin in April and May of 1991. I visited eight hospices, met their staffs, and interviewed both community physicians and surviving relatives of patients cared for by these hospices. I spent a day or more each at Hospice of the Bluegrass in Lexington, Hospice of Hope in Maysville, Hospice of Louisville, Lourdes Hospice in Paducah, and

Hospice of Central Kentucky in Elizabethtown, all in Kentucky; and HospiceCare in Madison, St. Joseph's Hospital Hospice Program in Marshfield, and Milwaukee Hospice Home Care, all in Wisconsin. I sat in on interdisciplinary team meetings, went along on intake visits, stayed overnight in the House of the Dove, a hospice residence in Marshfield, and had working lunches and dinners with groups of these hospices' staffs. I returned home with forty-two hours of taped interviews with sixty-five people. Most of the direct quotes in this book come from interviews done during that trip.

It is my experience that hospices do wonderful, inspired work with terminally ill patients and with their families, but the nature of that work can be so off-putting that it has led to a number of misconceptions about hospice care. Often people don't want to know about the reality of hospice until they really need it, and by then they are in a profound family crisis. I have tried to imagine the questions and concerns of people who might find themselves facing a decision about hospice care and to present the hospice experience within their frame of reference. I've tried to imagine what it must be like to confront such a decision, and what it really means to consent to a service designed expressly for the terminally ill. I've tried to describe what hospice care can offer to such people, and also to explain the limitations in what hospices can or will provide.

For some with life-threatening illnesses, deciding to enroll in hospice care will be an easy and obvious choice, because hospice is designed to address their very specific needs. For others, however, it must be a difficult and painful question, fraught with finality and grief— even when the support of hospice could be the best thing for dealing with their illness. The philosophy and the admission policies of hospices sometimes represent an emotional hurdle that is not easily surmounted until the illness has left them with no other choice. Sometimes it is just too hard for people to see themselves as appropriate for a program that cares for the dying — even when they are dying. However, families that have made it over this emotional hurdle to hospice care usually do not regret the decision.

Most of all, I have tried to emphasize that while hospice is care for the dying, it places a special emphasis on life and on living each day as fully as possible, with the hope of making the very best of today when your tomorrows are limited.

The great events of life, as we observe them, are still clearly
recognizable as journeys.... Out of centuries of experience has
come the repeated observation that death appears to be a process
rather than an event, a form of passage for human life.
— Sandol Stoddard,
The Hospice Movement: A Better Way of Caring for the Dying

The people who founded the modern hospice movement of humane care for the dying were guided by a few simple ideas. First, they believed that dying is a uniquely important time in a person's life. They viewed dying as the final stage of human existence and as a normal and natural process. But they also recognized that while death may be a natural process, it is rarely easy or simple. Hospice founders wanted to offer a specialized kind of support centered on the challenges unique to this process. They believed that care for the dying should involve a different pace and a different set of skills than other kinds of health care, with a primary emphasis on physical comfort and emotional support. They also believed that dying patients deserve to be informed about their medical condition and treatment alternatives, so they might make meaningful choices about how to live in the time remaining to them, and receive adequate care without having to feel demeaned or a burden.

Another observation of hospice founders was that the medical system frequently did not deal very well with the special needs of dying patients. In making this critique, they evoked another era in human affairs, when people tended to spend their lives surrounded by large, extended, multigenerational families. In earlier times the reality of death was harder to deny because it was closer to everyday life. The life cycle was played out for all to see, in nature, in agriculture, and in the family. People were born at home and died at home. While less-sophisticated medical care couldn't promise freedom from pain in those days, at least the extended family was present to offer caring and comfort. However, the growth of organized medicine and the development of modern medical institutions gradually changed all that, while a growing social mobility isolated many Americans from their families of origin. Responsibility for health care was turned over to doctors, and personal dramas of serious illness, once played out in the bosom of the family, were transferred to the hospital.

As a result, Americans today most often die in hospitals or other health facilities. We have come to place our faith in medicine, which has significantly extended human life spans through improved public health measures and seemingly miraculous new drugs and techniques, but when medicine fails to work its promised miracle, we feel betrayed.

The inability to arrest a disease also causes feelings of failure for doctors and for hospital staff — who are trained primarily in the practice of curative medicine and not in how to provide for a dying patient's comfort and emotional well-being. High-tech treatments, institutional routines, and an obsession with clinical test results tend to distance the doctor from the person who is terminally ill. Some doctors depend on emotional detachment to protect themselves from their own grief over the deaths of their patients. Terminal hospital patients might even be moved to the end of the ward, farthest from the nursing station, where they will not serve as a constant reminder of the system's failure. In these and other ways, the denial of an obvious terminal prognosis can leave the patient to die alone, in despair, fearful, angry, wracked with guilt, or in needless pain. (And for loved ones unspoken good-byes and unresolved grief are emotional time bombs that can wreak havoc years after.)

This was the reality that a number of Americans knew all too well when they first heard the English hospice physician Dame Cicely Saunders, the founder of the contemporary hospice movement, during her lecture tours of the United States in the early 1960s. Saunders was then in the process of creating the first true modern hospice, St. Christopher's, which opened in Sydenham in suburban London in 1967. In her American lectures, Saunders described her vision of a safe haven for the dying. Her concept of hospice was to combine the most modern medical techniques in terminal care with the spiritual commitment of the medieval religious orders that had once created hospices as way stations for people on pilgrimages. Saunders's new use of the word *hospice* evoked these original hospices, established throughout Europe. In the medieval hospices a link had been recognized between pilgrims on the perilous journey to the Holy Land and the dying, sojourners on an even more fearful and mysterious pilgrimage from this world to the next.

Medieval hospices evolved into institutions of spiritually inspired, loving care for the destitute, ill, and dying. Their tradition of service to "Our Lords the Sick" survived in a few outposts until Saunders and the modern hospice movement wedded it to modern techniques of pain relief, medical symptom management, and grief support for the terminally ill and for their families. For Saunders, the focus of the modern hospice movement began with attention to the nature of chronic terminal pain — the most feared manifestation of diseases such as cancer — and pain control has since remained the cornerstone of the hospice movement. Her message struck a responsive chord with Americans who knew from experience the need for such care, and with her inspiration they began the slow process of creating their own safe havens for the dying.

Some of these hospice pioneers were health professionals: doctors, nurses, social workers, counselors, or chaplains, frustrated with how impersonal medical technology and institutional routines could get in the way of their desire to truly care for dying patients. Others had lost a loved one to a disease such as cancer, and were either grateful for the care and support their loved ones received or else frustrated over lost opportunities and unrelieved suffering. America's hospice founders had also discovered that the human encounter with death, loss, and grief is one of the greatest opportunities in life for personal growth, self-insight, and spiritual understanding. These pioneers recognized the tremendous difference hospice could make in the lives of dying patients and grieving family members, and its ability to comfort, support, and empower those in need. In the nineteen years since the first American hospice, Connecticut Hospice, Inc., opened in New Haven, this powerful concept has spread to every state and to the establishment of sixteen hundred hospice programs nationwide, now serving two hundred thousand dying patients a year.

Through exposure to this new movement, the larger health care system has made significant advances in how it deals with terminal illness. Many health professionals now working in other settings have experience with hospice care, either directly or indirectly through making referrals to hospice programs. Hospice concepts of pain control today are more widely known and followed, and conspiracies of silence about terminal illness are less common. However, even today many people die in pain, denial, and isolation, often because they haven't heard of hospice or because the hospice option wasn't offered to them.

And new challenges in the 1990s make the hospice movement more important than ever. Advances in medical technology and public health that have significantly lengthened life spans have also led to an ever larger share of our population who are over sixty-five years of age — and especially over eighty-five. The longer people live, the more prone they are to degenerative illnesses such as cancer that hospice is designed to address. At the same time, the cost of health care has gone up dramatically in the past decade, reaching 12 percent of our gross national product, with a disproportional share of medical costs incurred during the last six months of life. In recent years the devastating epidemic of AIDS has created a new set of challenges for the health care system. Much of the system's current interest in hospice care is based on hospice's cost-effectiveness in caring for dying patients outside of the hospital while using less invasive, expensive medical technology. However, hospice's dramatic success in America has been driven even more by recognition of the humane alternative to conventional care it offers for the dying.

In her classic book *The Hospice Movement: A Better Way of Caring for the Dying,* Sandol Stoddard describes dying as a great journey and the modern hospice as "a place of meeting, a way station, a place of transit, of arrival and departure." The dying are going on ahead to where we all eventually must go,

Stoddard asserts. She traces the linguistic origins of the word *hospice* to the same root as that of our words *hostel, hospital* and *hospitality*: the Latin word *hospes*, meaning both host and guest. Stoddard also describes the rebirth of hospice as a haven and a caring community for the dying.

Today, our most common image of hospice care comes from the English prototypes such as St. Christopher's, where dying patients come to live out the remainder of their days in tastefully furnished, homelike settings. This image is understandable because it is easier to imagine hospice as a beautifully landscaped country house, far from where we live, where the terminally ill can "go to die." It may be harder to conceive of hospice's reality, but in the United States hospice care has developed primarily as a program or a philosophy of care, not a place to go. A coordinated team of hospice workers generally will come to you and care for you in your own home, rather than you going to them. Hospice is committed to doing everything in its power to help dying patients remain in their homes, cared for by family and friends with the expert support of health professionals and volunteers, until they die.

Sometimes it isn't possible for patients to remain in their homes, perhaps because the home is unsafe or inadequate, or the family is not present or able to participate in the care, or else medical symptoms are too complicated to be managed at home. For such situations many hospices have developed in-patient units for acute care and substitute home settings such as hospice residences or nursing home–based hospice units. But the basic thrust of hospice in America remains to provide care and support in the patient's own home, because for most people no substitute setting could ever be as familiar or reassuring as their own home.

With the advice and encouragement of hospice staff, families also discover that the responsibility of caring for a dying loved one at home can be successfully managed. Hospice provides the opportunity to make the most of precious time together, and helps families fulfill a dying loved one's wish to be at home rather than in a hospital or nursing home. And as family members gradually come to grips with their own grief and loss after a loved one's death, knowing what they were able to do for their loved one in those final days will be a great comfort.

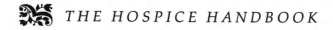 *THE HOSPICE HANDBOOK*

CHAPTER ONE

What Is Hospice Care?

I'd like people to understand that the whole purpose of the hospice program is to help. We judge our success on whether we've been able to help you. I hear people say to me, over and over, "We need some help." I would hope that any hospice anywhere would be a resource and a help to you. If you've got somebody with cancer in your family, call hospice — even if you don't know whether you're going to still pursue aggressive treatments. I don't mind taking a few extra phone calls.
— William Carter,
admissions coordinator, Lourdes Hospice, Paducah, Kentucky

Hospice is care for the dying. Its primary purpose is to work with the terminally ill and their families, to help them make the most of the time that's left, and to make their dying more comfortable, less frightening, and in every way more bearable. Hospice doesn't offer the prospect of cure or recovery to its patients, but when the disease can no longer be defeated, hospice proposes to help make the best of a hard situation.

The hospice approach has brought care and comfort to the lives of hundreds of thousands of dying Americans and their families. It offers an alternative to conventional, cure-oriented medical treatment aimed at fighting the disease by any means possible, at the time when that approach has

3

become counterproductive. For people with terminal cancer and other end-stage illnesses, the effects of futile, invasive treatments such as chemotherapy may be as harrowing as the disease itself. These harsh, powerful medicines that work by killing human cells — more of the abnormal cancer cells than healthy ones, it is hoped — eventually may add to, rather than diminish, the patient's suffering. At the same time the whirlwind of clinic visits, tests, treatments, and hospitalizations can stand in the way of trying to make good use of the time that remains. The mobilization of high-technology treatment to fight a serious illness can also limit the patient's control over his or her life, as the schedules and procedures of the medical system take precedence over the person's normal routines.

To the greatest extent possible, hospice tries to give back to its patients independence and control over the daily events of their lives. It asks questions: What does the patient really want and need at this point in his or her life? What might make the patient's day brighter and more meaningful? Decisions about schedules, treatments, meal plans, and visitors are returned to the patient and family, with expert guidance from hospice professionals about what can still be accomplished. Hospice also acts as an advocate for its patients and tries to help them sort out their real priorities.

Hospice provides palliative, or comfort, care, which means focusing on the relief of any discomforts caused by the illness, rather than attempting to cure the underlying disease. Hospice emphasizes quality of life, as that is defined by the patient, when quantity of life has become limited. With such an emphasis, hospice care tends not to include much aggressive, high-tech, cure-oriented medical treatment, except when such efforts can make a contribution to the patient's immediate comfort and well-being. Hospice care generally doesn't include heroic medical measures like cardiopulmonary resuscitation or other techniques that are used on an intensive care unit. The hospice philosophy essentially proposes to neither hasten nor postpone death's natural advance for a terminally ill patient, but instead to manage the patient's care as well as possible until the moment of death arrives. Thus, hospice care is not the same as active euthanasia, and hospices *do not* practice mercy killing or assisted suicide. Hospice workers are inspired by a reverence for life and respect for the individual, but they also believe in letting death come at its own pace, past the point where any heroic measures to stave it off can only have the effect of prolonging the patient's suffering and dying process.

Hospice aims to make its patients as pain-free, as alert, as comfortable, and as active as possible for as long as possible. This is achieved through careful attention to the little details that shape quality of life for the patient. Such attentive care requires careful assessment of the patient's needs by hospice staff, documentation of findings, continual reassessment, and thorough team planning to come up with effective solutions for each medical problem. Hospice is carried out under the basic guidance of a written plan of care for each patient, developed by the team of hospice professionals with frequent input by telephone from the patient's doctor, who retains medical responsibility for the patient's care.

For many hospice patients the first priority is the relief of their chronic, severe pain. By combining aggressive, around-the-clock use of opiate pain relievers such as oral morphine with complementary nondrug pain control techniques, hospices can often promise their patients that they will be pain-free within days of initiating hospice care. Hospice teams also use the most advanced medical techniques to relieve other distressing symptoms or discomforts of terminal illness, such as nausea, constipation, shortness of breath, or confusion.

Electric hospital beds, wheelchairs, bedside commodes, tub bars, and other adaptive medical devices are used to facilitate the patient's comfort at home. Patients may become too weak to leave their bed in the final weeks and will need hands-on assistance from the hospice personal care aide for bathing and toileting, as well as frequent changes of position and the use of egg-crate mattresses to prevent bedsores.

Once the patient's physical pain and discomfort are brought under control, attention can be shifted to other problems, such as family conflicts or fears and anxieties related to the impending death. Hospice social workers can help the patient and family deal with practical concerns: applying for insurance benefits, dealing with creditors, making wills, and planning for funeral arrangements. Personal estrangements or separations may be resolved with hospice's encouragement, leading to emotionally healing good-byes with family and friends. The hospice team also enlists the support of other available community resources when needed, including social services and disability coverage from the government, nutritional supplements from the American Cancer Society, counseling, and school tutors for children. When family resources are limited, hospice mobilizes additional bedside support from trained volunteers, neighbors, the patient's church or congregation, and the larger community.

Hospice also opens the door to talking about difficult issues. Hospice workers do not tell their patients how to die or force them to talk about death. Instead, they provide a sounding board, an opportunity, and a safe haven for patients to talk about whatever is most important to them — even subjects that family and friends are afraid to discuss. Hospice also suggests — contrary to some deeply held cultural reflexes in our society — that it's okay to talk openly and honestly about even the most tragic of circumstances. Sometimes, in fact, it's vitally important to talk about such painful realities, or else patients and families end up feeling even more isolated in their confusion and grief.

Our instincts sometimes tell us that if we just don't say out loud a bad word like "cancer" or "terminal," then somehow it won't turn out to be real. But the truth is, refusing to talk about it won't make it go away. Facing up to a bad reality isn't going to make it worse or cause it to happen sooner. In fact, if one can express deeply held fears and worries, some of them can be allayed — or at least their burden shared with others. Perhaps there are important matters that need to be taken care of, such as clearing up long-standing misunderstandings or planning for the family's financial future and children's upbringing. Once the painful reality is put on the table, it becomes possible to make realistic choices about one's life and to plan for contingencies.

Hospice workers have the experience to understand some of what the patient is going through. They also bring information to teach the family how to take care of the patient and deal with whatever might come up in the course of the illness. Hospice workers don't have any easy answers about what happens to us after we die, but they can help people air their questions and explore their own answers. With hospice's help people find they have sources of inner strength and ways of coping that they never realized they had.

Hospice also encourages patients to set and focus on current goals. These may include saying good-byes and summing up what one's life has meant, or just finding moments of peace or joy each day. People who are terminally ill can still be active participants in life. They may not always be bedbound or in need of supervision. They may be able to take trips to revisit a favorite park or restaurant. Even getting out of bed, into a wheelchair, and out of the sickroom may be an important psychological victory. Hospices sometimes suggest placing the patient's electric hospital bed in the living room, close to the center of family life; mounting a birdfeeder outside the window; providing a portable tape player with the patient's favorite music or inspirational messages; or encouraging the person to reminisce and reflect by looking through old photograph albums. Hospice care is about fully utilizing the life that remains to dying patients, about the choices that people can still make for their lives, about the meanings and values and relationships that can be emphasized despite a terminal illness.

❧ What Is a Hospice?

A hospice is a well-coordinated set of services intended to relieve or ease the varied symptoms or side effects of a terminal illness. Many hospices are community-based agencies created just for this purpose, while others are departments or units of hospitals or home health agencies, although such hospice departments have the same specialized focus on care for the dying. Hospice also refers to the concept or philosophy of care practiced by these specialized programs.

Hospice services are directed by a physician and planned and provided by a team composed of nurses, social workers, chaplains, therapists, personal care aides, and volunteers. Medical direction for the hospice team usually comes from the patient's primary physician, who in effect writes a prescription for hospice care, then reviews and authorizes the care the hospice provides. When needed, consultation is also provided by the hospice's medical director, a specialist in terminal symptom management.

Most of the services provided by a hospice can also be found in other corners of the health care system. The individual components of a hospice program aren't all that different from what might be offered by a home care agency, a public health nursing department, a hospital, a clinic, a nursing home, or any number of other health services that were providing care to people with life-threatening illnesses before hospice appeared on the scene. What's different about the hospice approach is its comprehensiveness, its specialization in the unique needs of the terminally ill, and the commitment to humane care for the dying that underlies everything a hospice does. The team of hospice professionals assumes case management responsibility for all the care a terminally ill patient needs.

Most of the time the actual care of a hospice is provided in the homes of dying patients, where the patient can be maintained in more comfortable, familiar surroundings, attended by family and friends. This care is blended with the family's routines as much as possible. Hospice is *not* a place where patients go to die: it is a service that comes to wherever the patient is living. Sometimes it is not possible for the patient to be cared for at home, and in those cases hospice programs try to provide alternative settings called hospice inpatient units, residential hospices, or nursing home–based hospice units. Thus, while hospice is a program, rather than a place, hospices may maintain substitute residences where patients can live when staying in their own home is no longer feasible.

Hospice inpatient units aim to be as homelike as possible, with flexible menus and eating schedules, twenty-four-hour visiting permitted for families, children, and even pets, and design features that soften the atmosphere of the institutional setting. At other times the hospice will send extra caregiving staff into the patient's home to function as family surrogates. As patients move between their homes and inpatient settings, hospice is also responsible for ensuring that consistency in their care continues without interruption. To hospice, home is wherever the patient happens to be living at the moment.

Hospice care in the home is typically provided on an intermittent basis, meaning that hospice staff are not present with the patient all day or all night, except in certain crisis situations. Instead, they come to the home for regularly scheduled visits to assess the patient's condition and needs, answer the family's questions, and address any practical concerns that have come up since the last visit. Hospice is also able to respond to emergencies in the home, with an on-call telephone system evenings and weekends when regular staff are not working. A nurse is available to field calls from hospice families twenty-four hours a day and, if necessary, to go to the home to help resolve crises.

Hospice tries to support the family's traditional strengths and coping skills in the face of a crisis. The "family" is defined broadly to include everyone who is personally important to the patient, whether legally related or not, including partners, lovers, friends, roommates, and neighbors. Hospice works closely with family members, educating and supporting them so that *they* can do most of the day-to-day, hands-on care of the patient. Families learn to participate directly in all aspects of the patient's care, to give scheduled medications and even to perform highly technical medical procedures — with the supervision and support of the hospice staff. They are also coached in what to expect as the patient's physical condition changes.

Hospice also pays attention to the family's needs and concerns, and supplements their efforts with extra help when that is needed. Hospice can provide them with breaks from their caregiving responsibilities by sending volunteers to the home or by placing the patient on the hospice inpatient unit for a few days, allowing caregivers to recover from pent-up stress or exhaustion. Hospice tries to help families gain confidence in their ability to cope with caregiving responsibilities and to know that they are giving their loved one the best care possible.

Hospice's care and caring do not cease when the patient dies. It has been recognized that the grief and loss people experience after the death of a loved one can themselves be significant health challenges. Hospice grief specialists support families during their bereavement for a year or more after the patient's death, helping them to understand the overpowering and confusing experience of grief, and encouraging them to tell the story of their loss — over and over again if necessary. Hospice tries to normalize the grief experience, helping people understand that they are not going crazy. Hospice bereavement support helps family members work through and resolve their grief until they are once again able to resume full and active participation in a world that has been forever altered by their loved one's absence.

Often families who start out believing they could never cope with the crisis of a terminal illness in their midst are gently supported and shown that they can manage, one day at a time. With hospice's help they are able to offer their dying loved one the opportunity to spend precious final days at home, usually without pain, and to play a very meaningful role in their loved one's care. Hospice can't take away the personal tragedy of a terminal illness, but it can make the experience more bearable for everyone involved.

🦋 *Beverly*

Beverly Thielman and her second husband, Don, married only six months, had just arrived in Madison, Wisconsin, where

Beverly was to start a new job with the Coalition of Wisconsin Aging Groups, when they found out Don had incurable melanoma. The discovery of the melanoma and a terminal prognosis were almost simultaneous, although Don was offered a potentially fatal new experimental treatment, which he refused. "He chose, in his independent way, that that would not be his course of action, and that allowed him to plan a different way of letting all this happen," Beverly explains. Don, not quite seventy, lived for a year with his illness, the last four months under the care of HospiceCare of Madison.

"Don's response to hospice was different than mine," she recalls. "We had just moved to this community, and my first thought was, I wonder if they have something like hospice that could help us. My husband's response was, 'We can do this ourselves.' But I knew I needed support. I just didn't know quite what that would be," she explains. "At that point, for him to say, 'Yes, we do need hospice care,' meant a lot of admissions, and it meant giving up a lot of his privacy and independence. But I think the personalities of the hospice nurse and social worker who came to our home and interviewed us convinced my husband that this was probably an okay thing to do after all. Meeting the HospiceCare people was all the reassurance I needed. They didn't march in and take over. They very compassionately, very gently introduced themselves, and they didn't intrude in our lives at all."

CHAPTER TWO

For Whom Is Hospice Intended?

You don't want to give up too early, but it's really great if you can be blessed with a sense of peace as you get closer to the end.
— John J. Gohmann, M.D.,
oncologist, Lexington, Kentucky

Most of the patients who enroll in hospice, and most of the hospice patients mentioned in this book, are people with cancer. Cancer refers to a group of diseases characterized by uncontrollable growth and spread of abnormal cells, which, if not checked, may end in death. According to the American Cancer Society, an estimated 1.1 million Americans were diagnosed with cancer in 1991, and about 514,000 died of the disease. Roughly half of those diagnosed with cancer today will survive their cancer for five years, at which point they may be considered cured. Thanks to continual improvements in research and in the screening and treatment of cancer, the cure rate keeps improving, slowly but steadily. However, cancer remains the number two overall cause of death for Americans, following heart disease.

Statistics show that actual cancer survival rates vary widely by the site and type of tumor and by how early it gets detected and treated. For example, breast cancer that is still localized at the time of diagnosis can be successfully treated 91 percent of the time. Prostate cancer can be cured 71 percent of the time, 85 percent if discovered while the disease is still localized. Colon cancer is 88 percent treatable and rectal cancer is 80 percent treatable if detected early. However, the five-year survival rate for lung cancer is only 13 percent, and only 3 percent of those diagnosed with pancreatic cancer will survive five years. Of course, these are very generalized figures. The patient's personal physician will have specific information about the individual's medical situation, disease progression, and prospects for recovery.

But what these numbers really mean is that while half of the people diagnosed with cancer today will get better, half won't make it, and for certain internal organ cancers the proportion who will fail to survive is much higher. Such people are the primary candidates for hospice care, once they have pursued and exhausted promising medical treatments recommended by their physicians. Approximately 84 percent of the 207,000 patients served by U.S. hospices in 1990 had cancer, according to the annual hospice census compiled by the National Hospice Organization. About one in every three Americans who died of cancer in 1990 received the support of hospice at the end of their lives.

Because of the preponderance of cancer patients among the clientele of hospices, the primary emphasis of hospice care in America has been on addressing the manifestations of terminal cancer. However, hospices also serve patients with other terminal diagnoses, including end-stage heart, lung, liver, or kidney disease, ALS (amyotrophic lateral sclerosis, or Lou Gehrig's disease), end-stage Alzheimer's disease and other neurological disorders, and AIDS (acquired immune deficiency syndrome). While many American hospices have served terminally ill AIDS patients with courage and compassion, some differences in their care from that of the typical hospice cancer patient have required a few modifications to the basic hospice approach in order to better meet their needs.

According to the National Hospice Organization census, two-thirds of hospice patients are over sixty-five years of age, and all but one percent are over eighteen. People over sixty-five, who are closer to the end of a normal human life span and who may feel they have already lived a full and productive life, are sometimes more receptive to a service such as hospice that emphasizes death as a natural part of life. However, the support and the expertise of hospice may be even more urgently needed when the dying patient is younger and less able to emotionally deal with his or her impending mortality. Many hospices will also serve children with life-threatening illnesses, and some have even developed specialized pediatric hospice services to address the different needs of families struggling to care for these children. The main concepts of hospice care can be applied, regardless of age or diagnosis, to anyone in need of a program of support targeted at the challenges of a terminal or life-threatening illness.

❧ Requirements for Enrollment in Hospice

1. *The patient has been given a medical diagnosis of a terminal illness, usually measured by a prognosis of six months or less left to live.* While most hospices require that the patient's prognosis be quantifiable in this way, some may extend the prognosis to a year, or else take a more flexible approach that doesn't specify a length of time. Instead, their policies may state that the patient should have a limited life expectancy, or an end-stage or life-threatening illness, or a disease not amenable to cure.

For many patients — and some physicians — the requirement of six months or less to live as a condition of hospice admission can be a barrier to using hospice. However, this requirement needs to be understood as it was intended: a best professional guess by the physician and a rough one at that. No one can accurately predict how long an individual will live with his or her disease. The best that can be done is an estimate based on how long people with a similar condition generally survive.

Hospices do not want to enroll patients too early — while they still have a chance for cure or might still benefit significantly from aggressive medical treatments. This is why hospices require the attending physician to certify that the patient in fact is terminally ill, with a life expectancy of six months or less to live — assuming that the illness continues to progress as anticipated. Medicare actually requires two physicians to certify that the patient has six months or less to live before that patient can qualify for the Medicare hospice benefit.

In reality, few patients come to hospice too early; more often they come very late, just days before they die. Hospice professionals find the latter situation harder to work with, because it is difficult for the hospice and for the family to deal with the dying process without adequate time to institute effective pain control measures or prepare for the tumultuous final days at the patient's bedside. Instead of good preparation for the death, they must resort to crisis management, which isn't satisfactory to anyone involved. American hospices tend to see patients during the last twenty to eighty days of their lives (on average fifty-nine days). This suggests that patients and their doctors, because of the hospice requirement of six months or less to live, may wait until the patient really only has days or weeks left to live before calling hospice.

Hospice's emphasis on the amount of time to live also

underscores the fact that hospice care is not designed for patients who have chronic long-term illnesses or are expected to live with their disease for years. The reason for this distinction is that hospice gears up to provide a more intensive level of care during the stressful terminal or end stage of illness. If a hospice program enrolled too many patients with chronic illnesses and years left to live, then its resources might not be available for the patients who needed it most, during the end stage. However, it would be a shame if families failed to investigate the hospice option simply because of the six-month requirement. In practice, most hospices try to be flexible and reasonable about this requirement and want to help you make the best decisions for your care.

2. *The patient is seeking comfort-oriented care, rather than treatment aimed at cure.* The underlying reason for this requirement is to clearly distinguish hospice as a program designed for those who are terminally ill and can no longer benefit from curative, aggressive treatment. Hospice provides palliative care, which promotes physical and emotional comfort for the patient when treatments aimed at cure are no longer realistic or appropriate. In practice, however, this distinction between palliative hospice care and curative treatment may not always be clear and easy to define.

Some hospices may have a list of medical treatments that are considered "hospice-appropriate" or else that are excluded from hospice coverage. Treatments to relieve the patient's pain — no matter how expensive or high-tech — are typically included in the hospice program, while experimental treatment protocols or certain surgeries, such as bone marrow transplants, typically would not be hospice-appropriate. Hospices also try to determine case-by-case whether a potentially aggressive therapy has a palliative intent for a patient. Since these can be difficult questions for patients and families, some hospices may enroll and work with the patient and family for several weeks in order to build up some trust, and then try to clarify what the patient and family really want. Once that becomes clear, some patients may decide to revoke their hospice enrollment in order to continue pursuing curative treatment. In other cases the hospice may agree to one last round of aggressive treatment in order to help a patient make the transition to the palliative approach.

3. *The patient and family are informed about hospice and other options, and consent in writing to hospice care; the patient's physician also consents to hospice.* Informed consent to medical treatment is a basic ethical and legal principle in our system of health care. Hospice tries to restore the patient's informed consent to treatment to its rightful importance. Hospices work hard to make sure that their patients know what the hospice philosophy and approach are all about, and that they are freely choosing it, before they enroll in hospice care. With any medical treatment there is the danger of miscommunication between provider and patient, inadequate exchange of information, or unmet expectations. With hospice care the danger is more serious, because hospice proposes to make the dying patient comfortable, but not to provide a medical cure. If that is not what the patient and family want, then serious disappointments or conflicts may follow. Often the hospice admission process explicitly states or implies that the patient should want to be maintained at home for as long as possible and that the family is willing and able to participate in the patient's care at home.

The concept of informed consent to hospice care can conflict with the desire of some families or doctors to shield patients from the reality of their medical condition. For purposes of admission requirements, hospices usually insist on the right to be honest with their patients about the general nature and focus of hospice care. They often also insist on being able to honestly answer patients' questions about their medical condition. Hospice believes that patients have a right to know the reality of their situation in order to make informed decisions about the limited life that remains to them. Hospice experience also suggests that conspiracies of silence to protect the patient from harsh truths usually don't work because the patient knows he or she is getting worse. However, hospice's emphasis on truthfulness does not mean that the patient must be brutalized with unwanted candor. The patient should have the right to say he or she doesn't want to hear certain painful facts, and serious medical information should be transmitted slowly and sensitively enough to allow the person an opportunity to do that.

Informed consent in hospice is achieved through an admission process and a written consent form that explain what hospice is, and by asking the patient and family their goals and what they already know about the illness. The admission interview may take an hour or more, and may even be spread over more than one session. However, because patients and families are likely to be in emotional turmoil, it may be necessary to revisit these questions over the coming weeks, to remind patients about what hospice is and what it does. Usually, a family member with primary responsibility for the patient's care witnesses the consent to hospice care and gives his or her own consent as well. The patient's physician, too, must be consulted, to confirm the patient's condition and terminal prognosis. The doctor also contributes to and approves the hospice's written plan of care for the patient, as well as any subsequent changes in treatment.

Hospice cannot admit the patient if the physician is opposed, so it may be necessary to discuss the hospice option with the physician and find out why he or she is opposed. If the patient is seeking a program of care for the dying, and the doctor doesn't believe the patient is terminally ill, obviously there is a misunderstanding somewhere. Sometimes patients need to be more direct in asking for information or a hospice referral from their physician, perhaps because the doctor feels they couldn't handle the truth or else is personally uncomfortable with issues of human mortality. Other times patients need to approach other health professionals, such as an office nurse or hospital social worker, to get the referral process started. Some doctors may be reluctant to work with hospice for other reasons. In extreme, rare cases where a patient really wants hospice but the physician is adamant, the patient may need to find another doctor willing to take over medical care responsibilities and to sign the hospice consent form. Although hospices are reluctant to come between patients and their physicians, in these extreme cases the hospice may be able to recommend another doctor to the patient.

It is to be hoped that the effort spent obtaining informed consent to hospice care from the patient, family, and physician is just the beginning of an open, collaborative relationship in which everyone involved contributes to the hospice plan of care and cooperates in making the care as successful as it can be, with success defined by the goals the patient and family have articulated. Informed consent thus should be an ongoing process, not just a one-time event. In a few cases, irreconcilable differences over goals or an inability to work together may become a problem, making it hard for the hospice to remain involved in the patient's care — perhaps even necessitating a mutually agreed upon discharge from hospice care.

4. *Hospice must be provided in a safe setting for care.* This requirement is defined in different ways by different hospices, but with the overall goal that hospice care is attempted under cir-

cumstances that are realistic and workable — such as a secure home environment with safe arrangements for hospice staff to visit the home and, usually, the presence of a family caregiver. Hospices often require that the patient have a family member or friend who is able and willing to act as primary caregiver in the home and participate actively in the hands-on care of the patient on a daily basis. However, the extent of this responsibility will vary from hospice to hospice and from patient to patient.

Since dying patients eventually lose the physical ability to safely care for themselves, and since hospice is not equipped to provide twenty-four-hour staffing or to supervise the patient's safety around the clock, admitting a patient who lives alone, with no family to help with the care, often becomes problematic. Also, if the patient should become comatose, confused, or otherwise unable to continue expressing his or her wishes regarding care, the hospice team will need to work with someone else who is responsible for the patient's welfare, such as a next of kin, best friend, or person designated with power of attorney.

The need for a safe home setting and a willing family caregiver can be a frustrating requirement, since patients who live alone often need hospice's care and support even more than those who have family members participating in their care. At one time, most American hospices reluctantly turned away patients who lived alone and had no family or friends willing to take an active role in their care. Recognizing how unfair it was to turn away such patients, hospices are now experimenting with ways to accommodate them. This may be done by mobilizing shifts of friends, neighbors, volunteers, and others from church or community groups to fill a care schedule in the patient's home. Hospices may come to an agreement with patients specifying that when they are no longer able to remain at home safely, they will consider other options, such as hiring their own live-in helper or going into a nursing home.

Some hospices are also developing contractual relationships with nursing homes so that they can bring the spirit and expertise of hospice care into the nursing home setting for terminally ill nursing home residents. Others have opened residential programs that provide homelike, noninstitutional settings where dying patients can live out their remaining days when staying at home is no longer possible. Despite these alternatives, about 40 percent of U.S. hospices still require the presence of a family caregiver in the home as a condition of admission to hospice services, according to the National Hospice Organization.

5. *A do-not-resuscitate order.* Another requirement for admission to some hospice programs is that the patient elect a do-not-resuscitate (DNR) order, meaning that the patient — and the patient's doctor — agree in advance that no cardiopulmonary resuscitation (CPR) or other heroic measures will be attempted if the patient's heart should stop beating. This, too, can be an emotional hurdle for patients and families, since it is yet another reminder that the patient is terminally ill and not expected to recover. However, hospices believe that aggressive cardiopulmonary resuscitation is an inappropriate, invasive treatment for patients who already have end-stage cancer or other terminal illnesses, since it merely prolongs the dying process without offering much hope for regaining meaningful quality of life. They may also feel that requiring a DNR order helps to clarify whether or not the patient is emotionally ready for the hospice approach. Other hospices may require patients to be willing to discuss and clarify their wishes relative to resuscitation, whichever course they then choose. Hospices also try to educate patients and families about the

consequences of attempting resuscitation on a patient who is already terminally ill.

However, requiring a DNR order as a condition of admission may no longer be permitted under the Patient Self-Determination Act which went into effect in December of 1991. This law requires hospices and other federally funded health care providers to inform their patients about their rights under state law to refuse medical treatments or to initiate advance care directives such as a living will or Durable Power of Attorney for Health Care. The new law clearly prohibits discrimination against patients based on whether or not they have executed an advance directive. What is not clear is whether a DNR order should be considered an advance directive for purposes of this law. In some ways a DNR order resembles other routine medical orders for a patient's care signed by a doctor, but at the same time it involves formalized planning for future life-and-death eventualities, just like an advance directive. Federal guidelines for implementing the Patient Self-Determination Act have left it up to each state to formulate its own definitions of advance directives. If the state considers DNR to be an advance directive, as some states do, then it follows that hospices in that state cannot require a DNR order as a condition for receiving their services. However, this does not mean that the hospice is required to *provide* resuscitation to its patients. The patient and family, in giving informed consent to hospice care, need to acknowledge that they understand the hospice does not provide CPR. The family would be acting on their own if they decided to call 911 or other emergency medical services when the patient's heart stops.

6. *Other admission requirements.* Individual hospices may use other admission requirements reflecting local resources and needs. Most hospices, for instance, have clearly defined geographical service boundaries, since hospice staff must travel

to the patient's home. Hospices are always expanding to serve more territory, but there are still areas that do not have access to hospice services. These tend to be isolated rural areas or communities that are medically underserved. Other hospices may limit their services to a specific population group, such as beneficiaries of a health maintenance organization or health insurance plan, or armed services veterans receiving medical care at a Veterans Administration hospital. Some hospices, recognizing limits to their specialized expertise, also limit their service to patients with cancer or to adult patients, although this approach is becoming rare. Hospices may also refuse to get involved in a family situation where there is active alcohol or drug abuse by the patient or family members, or where other circumstances make care at home difficult or unsafe for hospice staff.

﷽ *Grace*

Grace (not her real name), interviewed a year after her husband, Bill, died at home under the care of a Wisconsin hospice, says, "Bill's doctor was instrumental in inspiring me to call hospice, but he mentioned it several times before I actually got around to calling. I don't think Bill ever really knew what hospice was. I was the one who benefited from hospice and from the fact that Bill was being cared for by absolutely wonderful people and that his physical needs were being taken care of. Then these young women would come and sit down with me and talk about what was happening to me in my everyday life. I was just enchanted by that, and very comforted," she says. "The way you feel when your husband is ill, you know, your stomach is churning, you're a nervous wreck, you don't eat very well, you don't sleep for beans. So you need somebody... to tell you what to do, to help you make decisions, and I liked that part very much."

How difficult was it for Grace to care for her husband? "I was terrified every time I brought him home from the hospital. I always felt totally inadequate," she says. "Then hospice came along. That was very comforting to me, but I still was an absolute wreck." A friend drew up a chart with the schedule for Bill's various medications, while hospice staff demonstrated the use of a draw-sheet system on his bed that made it easier for Grace and her daughters to move him. "One bit of advice they gave me that was absolutely wonderful was to put the hospital bed in the library, on the first floor, right in the middle of things. I slept on the davenport at that time so I'd be close when he called me in the middle of the night," she says. "And then when he needed oxygen, it was just like somebody took a wand and waved it over my head, and the oxygen magically appeared."

One night Grace had to change Bill's oxygen tank because the one in use was nearly empty. "I called up the hospice and a nurse there said, 'Now, just relax, you're going to be all right. I'll walk you through this.' That kind of thing, it was absolutely marvelous — their ability to be sensitive to what might be on your mind. One afternoon two of the women from hospice came by. They sat and visited with me for a short period of time. Bill was dozing. And then the nurse pulled her chair up to mine and said, 'You realize that Bill is showing all of the symptoms of approaching death.' She had a mimeographed sheet, and we checked each thing off. They did it very deliberately, very caringly, but that was very revealing. I think it was then that I called my children and told them to come home."

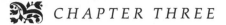

CHAPTER THREE

The Services Provided by a Hospice

> *Patients and families tell us we do something that nobody else is willing to do — to be present with them at a hurtful, hateful, raw time in their lives, and to be comfortable in being there, and not just standing by, but really rolling up our sleeves and getting in there to help.*
> — Elaine Cox
> *director, Lourdes Hospice, Paducah, Kentucky*

The American hospice movement began in part as a consumer movement, as an attempt to fill a perceived need or lack in the health care system for consumers who had terminal illnesses. Potential clients of hospice care should be informed consumers, and have a right to ask what kinds of benefits enrolling in a hospice program might bring them. "I guess we don't talk about this much, but the product of hospice — what we really do — is help people face death and come to some kind of comfort level with that," says Norman McRae, the director of Hospice of Hope in Maysville, Kentucky. "Hospice aims to help people find some quality time and, even though they're dying, to look at the miracles that can still happen in the days they have left."

"Hopefully," adds William Carter, of Lourdes Hospice in Paducah, "somewhere along the way the patient gets to some point where he can accept the fact that, 'Hey, I'm not going to get better, and, therefore, I have to pack a lifetime of living into whatever time I have left.' And that really is the thrust of all our jobs in hospice: how can we help that patient in the days that he has left?"

Although hospices can't guarantee 100 percent success in relieving the pain and other symptoms of a terminal illness, they aggressively pursue medical symptom management, and succeed very often. Hospices also aim to offer their patients options and choices throughout the dying process. Hospice professionals act as patient advocates, reminding patients that they have the right to make choices about their medical care. Often just giving information and clear explanations of what's happening to the person and of what's still achievable can be empowering. Patients may feel intimidated by their doctors and reluctant to ask hard questions or to have confusing information repeated or explained. Hospice staff can help patients sort out what their questions really are, write them down before the next appointment, and make sure they get answered by the doctor. Hospice teaches that it's okay to ask why: Why am I having this treatment? What are its benefits? Does this test or treatment simply satisfy the doctor's curiosity, or will it make a meaningful contribution to my life?

Hospice also offers advice and troubleshooting in anticipation of the common crises likely to come up in the course of the illness, with an emphasis on preparedness throughout the dying process. Hospice aims to provide solutions for all of the problems related to a terminal illness, whether they are physical, social, psychological, emotional, practical, or spiritual in nature. "It can seem so overwhelming all at once," says Chris

Hughes, a social worker with Hospice of Hope in Maysville. "It can be such a help to just talk through these issues one at a time."

When the patient's death draws near, no matter what the hour, a hospice professional will be available to sit at the bedside with the family, offering them gentle encouragement and support. If they don't know how to act around a person who's dying or what to say, hospice can provide a positive example. Hospice staff may also encourage family members to just sit with a newly deceased patient's body for as long as they wish, rather than immediately calling a funeral home to remove the body. Some families may even wish to bathe the body as a sort of ritual farewell. It is best if, with hospice's encouragement, a choice of funeral parlor or cremation society and plans for a memorial or funeral service have already been made, so that family members don't have to grapple with these questions in their acute shock and grief. Other families might be more comfortable if the actual death takes place someplace else. In such cases the hospice may transfer the patient to its inpatient unit for the final few days.

Hospice also emphasizes the opportunity to die without a lot of the tubes, needles, bells, monitors, and other paraphernalia of high-technology medicine. Such technology can dehumanize the experience of dying and place physical and emotional barriers between the patient and loved ones at a time that could be the most intimate and powerful experience of their lives. A quieter, calmer, hospice-supported death at home can leave family members with a very different set of memories than the conventional experience of death on an intensive care unit.

"We're walking down a path with these people, and we let them know they don't have to walk it alone," says Lin Edwards, director of patient and family services for Hospice of Louisville, Kentucky. "We can only go so far down that path, but we're not going to abandon them." Adds Elaine Cox, "Hospice is almost like a guide . . . through the death process. Not one that's out in front of you saying, 'C'mon, this is the way to go.' And not someone who's back behind you pushing and saying, 'Let's get on with this.' But a guide who's standing right beside you, wherever you are in the journey, and whichever direction you choose to take. But a guide nonetheless, who can say to you: 'This is all right,' or, 'This is where the path is leading us.' That is what's so wonderful about hospice, because the end result to the patient and family is that you may have made it the best trip it can possibly be — even though this is the most difficult, heart-wrenching, terrible time in a person's life."

Hospices also emphasize closure, which means that to the extent possible everything important was said, everything necessary was done, and everything essential was resolved before the patient's death. Closure, says Sharla Dreikosen, social worker with St. Joseph's Hospital Hospice Program in Marshfield, Wisconsin, is "when both the patient and family feel that all is said and done, whether verbally or nonverbally. It's saying good-bye, or saying, 'I'm going to miss you, but I'll be okay.' The dying patient needs to hear that. A lot of times hospice helps the patient to know, 'My family is going to be okay, because hospice isn't going to forget about them,'" Dreikosen explains.

"Ultimately, a positive outgrowth of hospice care could be a family member's own growth and development through this whole process — through the end of their own grief," says Barbara Bouton Schmitt, director of volunteers and bereavement for Hospice of Louisville. "That's not a goal I would articulate to someone who's in the throes of this experience, because I don't think they can have the vision to see that down the road this could become a process of growth for them. But that is certainly something we've seen here in a number of family members who have been involved in our bereavement program. They say, 'You know, I never would have done something like that while my husband was alive,'" Schmitt explains. "They become whole again, in a different way. They are a different person than they were."

"I see hospice as having a presence and an accessibility that is not available elsewhere, for the most part," adds Rachel Yaron, head nurse for St. Joseph's Hospice in Marsh-field. "Until you're in the process of trying to work through the issues that dying generates, you don't know what your needs are. So by having that presence we can assist people in looking at the issues we found other patients and families had to work through," she explains.

Obviously, people were dying of cancer before hospice appeared on the scene, and many families today are coping with a terminal illness without the benefit of hospice. "I think people can probably do it themselves, without hospice," says Kate Ford Roberts, former clinical liaison nurse with Hos-piceCare in Madison, Wisconsin. "But the difference is that people feel nurtured, they feel cared for and affirmed in what they are doing — which gives them the strength to continue to care for that person. Yeah, they could do it by themselves, but at what emotional and physical cost?"

"Often there's a message we give to families," says Viola Runnion, director of social services for Hospice of Louisville: "'This is something you all may want to think about doing, simply because you're going to feel better if you do it. Later, when you look back on it, you're going to know you took the time and trouble and made the effort.' Sometimes they follow that advice, and later they say, 'I'm so glad we did.'" Lin

Edwards explains, "They can stand at that casket and say: 'I did everything I wanted to do. I gave my loved one a choice. I said everything I wanted to say. Our relationships were healed, even though the disease did not get healed.'"

🦢 *The Hospice Team*

The glue that holds together this hospice approach to care is the interdisciplinary team. The team meets regularly, often weekly or bi-weekly, to develop, maintain, review, and implement a written plan of care and treatment for each of the hospice's patients. Team members work closely together, aiming for a group consensus. Unlike various other types of teams, which usually have a boss or leader who dictates to the other members, in hospice much effort goes into making sure the team is truly participatory and inclusive. For most patients, the primary nurse acts as the focal point for hospice services, but since nobody can have all the answers, the nurse looks to other team members for guidance and to test his or her conclusions. The hospice medical director, a specialist in the management of symptoms of terminal illness, also provides expert advice and direction to the team.

The hospice team meeting combines highly technical medical discussions and suggestions with a discussion of team members' work; it also provides a forum for them to air their own grief when patients die. Sometimes it is important for the team to see how each different professional discipline has its own perspective and a different piece of the solution to a patient care problem. Some patient problems are very concrete, requiring the best techniques of symptom management. Others are much more ambiguous — important to the patient but with no obvious solution. While hospice's goal is to relieve the symptoms of terminal illness, in reality not all problems have resolutions, at least not in the short time hospice has to work. Thus, hospice team members also need to remind each other of their limits.

Documentation of everything that happens in hospice — including assessments done in the home by hospice staff, discussions at team meetings, discharge summaries from hospitals, communications with physicians, signed consent forms, and patients' advance directive documents, such as living wills — is essential to ongoing coordination and to the continuity of care provided by the team. When one team member is off work for vacation or illness, someone else will need to pick up where the care left off. All of this information ends up in a clinical chart securely stored in the hospice office, accessible to the on-call nurse for use in after-hours emergencies.

The hospice team also aims to maximize the number of visits to the patient's home each week by sending different professionals on different days. But there is bound to be a certain amount of overlap and blurring of professional roles because of the unpredictability of the illness. "In hospice, when you go into the home, you have to be a little bit of everything," says Chris Hughes. "The team concept says that there are a variety of approaches or different orientations or ideas that can make living with a terminal illness easier or better or help families cope in healthier ways," adds Barbara Bouton Schmitt. With the hospice team, "the whole is greater than the sum of its parts. Each person lends their own area of expertise, and that has value, but it's the whole together that really makes things work. The team sort of molds itself to the case," Schmitt explains. "I see the hospice team as being really fluid and flexible and open, so that the patient and family can redefine it in each case."

THE NURSE

The nurse plays a pivotal role in the care provided by the hospice team, serving as case manager or team captain for his or her patients, and coordinating the services of other team members. A hospice nurse working full-time may serve as case manager for anywhere from seven to fourteen dying patients and families, depending on the agency's structure, driving distances between homes, and the patients' intensity of need. Nurses plan and carry out their own schedules and are responsible for visiting every patient on their caseload on a regular basis, usually at least once a week, more often when necessary. Between visits, frequent telephone contact is maintained with the family.

The nurse's responsibility is for the total patient — for all of the needs or issues important to this person related to the terminal illness. However, the nurse's primary focus is on the patient's physical condition and comfort. The nurse must be in close communication with the patient's physician, acting as the doctor's eyes and ears in the home, because the patient's ability to visit the doctor's office is limited, while few physicians today enjoy the luxury of making home visits. The doctor must rely on the nurse's accurate observations and professional judgment to stay informed on the patient's progress. The nurse also confirms clinical findings and recommendations with the doctor, and reconciles current observations of the patient's condition with the doctor's knowledge of the patient's medical history.

The foundation of hospice nursing care is the skilled assessment, a formalized process that nurses are well trained to perform. The assessment basically starts at the head and goes right down the body, covering every organ system, with extra attention to known or suspected problem areas. Using hospital discharge information and the initial hospice assessment as a baseline, the nurse might measure heart rate, blood pressure, and body temperature, as well as listening to lung sounds, asking about the patient's pain and discomfort, and reviewing the schedule of medications. A physical assessment may also look at skin condition and skin breakdowns (bedsores), other troubling symptoms, such as edema (fluid build-up in the extremities), and the patient's concerns related to confusion, forgetfulness, insomnia, or anxiety. Hospice nurses also emphasize careful monitoring of the gastrointestinal tract and the potential for problems such as appetite loss, nausea, vomiting, diarrhea, constipation, or bowel obstruction. As with its other concerns, hospice tries to take a preventive approach to bowel care and eating problems. Not every aspect of a full physical assessment is done on every visit.

Physical symptoms of pain and discomfort are often intimately connected to the patient's emotional state and to other issues in the family. For example, fear, anxiety, or family commotions can make the patient's experience of pain worse. The hospice nurse must be a sensitive and attentive listener, recognizing that when it comes to the actual symptoms of illness the most reliable source of information is what the patient says. With symptoms such as pain, only the patient can say whether pain is present, how severe it is, how much of an impact it is having on daily life, and whether medical treatments are having any effect.

Since the family is doing much of the day-to-day care, another major responsibility for the hospice nurse is to educate family members on how to perform many of the basic care functions. These may involve catheters and intravenous lines, medication schedules and administration, the use of other medical equipment, simple dressing changes and skin care, mouth care, feeding, body mechanics, and transfers from bed to commode to wheelchair and back. The hospice nurse reinforces and monitors the family's progress in learning these essential tasks.

Another important responsibility for hospice nurses is providing emergency on-call coverage evenings and weekends, when the rest of the hospice team is off duty. Hospices employ answering services to screen their telephone calls after hours, and at least one nurse is always accessible by phone or pager to respond to medical emergencies or other serious crises in the patient's home at any time, day or night. Often the family's medical questions can be answered over the telephone, but if necessary, the nurse will go to the home to resolve the problem in person, or to attend at the patient's death. Typically the patient's physician — or a colleague acting as a stand-in — and the hospice medical director are also available by pager twenty-four hours a day for emergencies, but the first line of response is the on-call nurse.

THE SOCIAL WORKER

The hospice social worker provides what is called psychosocial support, which is a broad term covering the patient's emotional life, any past or present psychological problems, and all of the people in the patient's life: immediate family, distant relatives, friends, neighbors, co-workers, insurance companies, creditors, and many others. If the hospice nurse's primary focus is on the patient's comfort and all of the physical and emotional factors that impact on comfort, the social worker's arena is the patient's environment and relationships. A large part of the social worker's job is based on the logistics of hospice care and daily life with a terminal illness: how to apply for insurance benefits, Social Security, Medicaid, food stamps, or social service chore workers and how to deal with financial issues, wills, legal questions, or funeral planning. Social workers also know about other community services that may be available to disabled persons.

At times the social worker may become involved in supportive or therapeutic counseling for the patient or family, but again the focus is on practical, immediate issues such as family conflicts or fears and anxieties about the death. If there are significant, long-standing problems — such as alcohol or drug addiction, unresolved past grief, or family abuse issues — and if these problems are affecting the patient's care and quality of life today, the hospice social worker may recommend more in-depth counseling or refer the patient and family to a psychological specialist. Stressful situations such as caring for a terminally ill relative have a way of bringing up unresolved problems related to a previous death, loss, or separation. Generally, however, hospice philosophy recognizes that while the emotional pain and suffering related to terminal illness, death, and loss are very real, they are also very normal, not evidence of a psychological condition. Nor is the crisis of a terminal illness the best time to make major changes in the family. People cope with dying or with loss as they have coped with crises throughout their lives.

Soon after, or simultaneous with, the nurse's first home visit, the social worker will do an assessment of the family's psychosocial needs and ability to care for a dying patient, in order to identify "issues that will come up that might make the care harder," explains Olivia Burr, social worker with Lourdes Hospice. Burr describes the job as working with the various family members, "who may have all kinds of different information and rights and feelings about the dying process, and then I try to help them come to a consensus. It's almost like a negotiation," she adds. "My job is to make sure that they have all the resources necessary to take care of that patient." A common technique used by the hospice social worker is to convene a family conference, in which the people involved in the patient's life and care meet to air, discuss, and resolve their conflicts, disagreements, and misunderstandings in order to get everyone working together for the patient's needs.

"Sometimes we will find a whole grocery sack or a drawer or a shoe box full of unopened correspondence from medical providers and insurance companies," Hospice of Louisville's Viola Runnion relates. "There may be thousands of dollars' worth of insurance claims checks that have never been opened because the family just got stressed and overwhelmed. They don't know what to do with the bills and don't know how they're going to pay them and don't understand anything about it. So they just don't deal with it, and put it all out of sight. Our social workers will go through this pile at the family's request, and open all that stuff and sort it out and begin to see what's what and what needs to be done now."

PERSONAL CARE AIDE

The personal care aide is known by various job titles, including home health aide, homemaker, attendant, nurse's aide, or chore worker, depending on the source of reimbursement or payment for the aide's services, length of shift, and nature of services provided. The role of the home health aide in the patient's home is similar to the work of the nurse's aide in a hospital or nursing home, since the most basic care needs of people physically unable to take care of themselves are pretty much the same, whatever the setting.

The aide provides personal care assistance with the activities of daily living — tasks that most of us perform for ourselves every day without a second thought but that loom large when we are unable to care for ourselves. These include bathing, grooming, mouth care, hair care, skin care, assistance getting in and out of a bed or wheelchair, help in getting to the bathroom, turning and repositioning in bed, and housekeeping chores. Many of these tasks will be performed by the family, but some family members are limited in what they can do by their own physical impairments or by other responsibilities such as work or child care. The aide's participation in chores such as shopping, cooking, changing bed linens, laundry, and straightening out the patient's room will depend on how much the family is able to do, but with the recognition that a bedbound patient shouldn't have to go very long without attention to such basic needs as meals, bathing, or dry sheets. Also, family members may find it difficult or even somewhat repugnant to deal with certain bodily functions, such as bathing the patient's privates, tending to colostomy equipment, changing dressings on serious wounds, or cleaning up after bladder accidents, diarrhea, or vomiting.

To the hospice personal care aide, none of this is difficult or repugnant. Aides have basic training in all aspects of physical care, in body mechanics, and in the common manifestations of illness. They are also well trained in the universal infection control techniques now recommended for the care of all patients by the federal Centers for Disease Control. They bring to their work a philosophy of rolling up their sleeves and doing whatever needs to be done to make sure that the patient is managed safely and comfortably at home. Typically aides visit one to three times a week for up to two hours or more per visit. Direction comes from the nurse case manager and from the family, but the aide often spends more time than any other hospice team member in the patient's home, right at the patient's side. Because of the direct, intimate, hands-on nature of their work, aides may develop close personal relationships with patients and hear secrets that no one else on the hospice team hears. Giving a bed bath to a person who is

confined to bed or cheerfully cleaning up after a bowel accident can be an extremely intimate act. The manner in which
the aide performs these tasks is important, and the aide's role
also emphasizes companionship and emotional support.

"There's something about touching patients, putting
your hands on them, that opens them up to the aide more than
to anyone else on the team," says Stephen Connor, former coordinator of the Kaiser Permanente Hospice in Walnut Creek,
California. For patients and families who have chosen comfort-oriented hospice care at home rather than curative medical treatment in a hospital setting, the personal care aide may
be the most eagerly anticipated and deeply appreciated service that hospice provides.

THE HOSPICE CHAPLAIN

The belief that spiritual care is also essential for dying
patients and their families — and that it should be intimately
personalized, not just a formal visit from a clergyperson — is
fundamental to hospice philosophy. However, hospices vary
widely in the specifically spiritual care services they offer.
They also vary in terms of who is formally assigned to spiritual care responsibilities, and the title for this role: chaplain,
spiritual caregiver or coordinator, pastoral care worker, psychosocial counselor, or clergy representative. Many hospices
have paid staff filling this role, while others utilize a rotating
or on-call group of volunteer clergy from the community.
Hospice spiritual care providers may counsel patients directly, or else concentrate on identifying, contacting, and
working with the patient's priest, minister, or rabbi — or finding someone from the community for the patient who has no
current relationship with a clergyperson but now wants one.

While some hospices are sponsored by religious groups,
or else by hospitals with religious affiliations, all hospices are

firmly committed to being nonsectarian and nondenominational in the care they provide. There may be some confusion or apprehension about this by patients and families, who expect that the hospice chaplain will fill a primarily religious role, like the family minister. In fact, the chaplain aims to be of service to the patient's spiritual needs, whatever they are and however the patient chooses to define and understand them.

Hospices would never knowingly send out a representative who intends to encourage a deathbed conversion, urge repentance, or proselytize for any religious belief. Hospice professionals do not stand in judgment on their patients, regardless of circumstances, nor try to make them feel guilty or frighten them with apocalyptic visions of what awaits after death. Hospice believes that terminal illness is a time for forgiveness, healing, and acceptance. But if the patient asks for someone to represent his or her religion and what it says about death, or wants help in rediscovering old religious traditions that have gotten lost along the way, hospice can assist in this quest.

Hospice's commitment to spiritual care is addressed first of all through a spiritual assessment that at the very least asks such questions as: "Do you belong to a church or congregation?" "Does your minister know about your illness?" "Would you like us to contact your minister?" "Would you like a visit from the hospice chaplain?" In some hospices the spiritual care provider tries to visit each patient at least once, while in others the chaplain only visits if the patient requests it. For many dying patients and their families, religious perspectives, beliefs, and rituals are important sources of comfort. Bringing the sacraments to a patient's bedside, reading and discussing scriptural passages, and praying together are just some of the services hospice chaplains can provide directly or arrange for. They can also help explain the patient's spiritual concerns to the rest of the hospice team, and represent the hospice philosophy to community clergy.

Hospices also help patients deal with those spiritual concerns that aren't fully addressed through formal religious observances. Although dramatic deathbed conversions are not common in hospice, dying patients have many questions and fears. They may not even be able to articulate spiritual yearnings that they nonetheless feel very deeply. For hospice spiritual caregivers, it's important to be open to the patient's concerns and able to support the patient's struggles with questions that lack easy resolutions. In fact, the questions, the dialogue, and the spiritual companionship may be more important to the patient than finding absolute answers. Hospice of Louisville's chaplains, for example, define their role in terms of four fundamental spiritual needs found in every dying patient: the need to reflect on the meaning of life, the need to tell one's life story, the need for belonging and community, and the need for hope.

"We're all obligated to the spiritual side of hospice, in order to be guides and companions," says Elaine Cox. "Whether you're the nurse or the social worker or the pastoral counselor, you have to share your own spiritual sense. And I'm not saying you go in and talk to them about God. I'm saying that you go in and give them the opportunity to think about what this is that's going on with them and how it's impacting on them: 'What do you think about when you really think about where you're headed?'" Hospice believes that every person has a spiritual side, Cox adds. "We believe that should they want to, they should be able to express their spiritual side in a very nonthreatening environment. And expressing it can mean anything that the patient wants it to mean."

THE PATIENT CARE VOLUNTEER

The patient care volunteer's role in hospice might be summed up in two words: everything else. Hospice attracts and utilizes trained volunteers in a number of different roles, such as answering the telephone or helping with clerical tasks in the office, staffing the hospice thrift store or weekly bingo game, serving on the board of directors or on governance and advisory committees, running errands, and providing specialized services such as massage therapy, yardwork, or hairdressing for patients.

Many American hospices were founded by volunteers and depended in their early days on volunteers for virtually everything they did, including the medical and nursing care. As they grew and evolved, distinctions developed between paid hospice staff, who had defined professional roles, and lay volunteers, whose contributions were less clearly defined. Volunteers have a different motivation for their work than do even the most committed of paid staff, and people who volunteer to spend their free time with dying patients and families often draw on either personal experiences or some fairly serious thinking about meanings of illness, dying, and mortality.

The most common assignment for patient care volunteers is to work with a single hospice patient and family for the duration of the illness and perhaps significantly beyond, until a different team of hospice bereavement volunteers becomes involved. Volunteers may visit one to three times a week, for periods ranging from half an hour to half a day. At first, the volunteer's relationship with the patient and family is defined by specific practical chores or contributions the volunteer can make. It may evolve into something closer and warmer, akin to a friendship — but with the understanding that the volunteer is only there to help and to make the family's situation easier to manage. If the volunteer is no longer contributing in this way, then his or her presence in the home should be reevaluated.

Volunteers deliver medications, drive patients to the doctor's office, bring spouses to the supermarket, shovel snow or rake leaves, walk the patient's dog, take younger children on fun outings, take the patient to a restaurant for lunch, or read aloud to patients who can no longer read for themselves. If the patient needs to be attended, the volunteer can do that, allowing the family caregiver to get away for shopping, a haircut, a movie, or just freedom for a few hours from taxing responsibilities. A volunteer may play checkers with the patient, rent and watch a movie on the VCR, or even just sit quietly at the bedside while the patient sleeps. But more than anything the volunteer talks with patients and families, listening and participating in conversations about whatever they wish to discuss.

"One of our volunteers described her approach to each new family as going out to them as an unmolded lump of clay, and allowing them to mold her in the way that they needed her to be," says Hospice of Louisville's Barbara Bouton Schmitt. "Most of the requests we get are for those kinds of sitting things, sitting with the patient so the wife can do whatever it is she wants to do," she adds. "Some caregivers will just putter around the house or take a nap. Others have a Bible study group every Wednesday morning, or the wife gets her hair done every Friday at 10 A.M."

Some hospice families know exactly how a volunteer could help them or what they want done. Others are unclear as to why a volunteer would choose this line of work or how to use the volunteer. Hospice professional staff may point out specific practical tasks that the volunteer could do, reminding them that they don't have to have the volunteer back if they don't want to. Families should also know that volunteers are carefully screened by the hospice, in recognition that only someone with maturity and self-awareness can handle the responsibility. Hospice volunteer applicants who want to do missionary work with dying patients, or who have personal problems they hope to work out with their patients' help, will be steered in other directions.

Patient care volunteers are well trained, with up to thirty hours of intensive instruction in hospice philosophy, patient care concerns, communication skills, and the limits to the volunteer's role. Volunteers are also carefully supervised by the hospice team and the volunteer coordinator. They meet with other volunteers for regular peer support, talk frequently with the volunteer coordinator about their assignments, and are prepared for the fact that the patient's death may be a significant and painful loss for them, too. Volunteers are also encouraged to take breaks from hospice work and to seek out meaningful personal support for dealing with those losses.

"These are people who have successfully grasped the concept that death is part of a process or continuum in life," says Janet Clyde, former volunteer coordinator for Vesper Hospice in San Leandro, California. "Hospice volunteers are remarkable people. I have so much respect for them. They never miss a stride — they keep walking steadily over the steep parts and over the sad parts. I think there must be a terrific emotional payback from hospice. I think it must be the biggest high there is in volunteering."

OTHER TEAM MEMBERS

The patient's primary physician certifies the patient's terminal prognosis, consents to hospice care, approves the written plan of care and any subsequent changes, and continues to participate through telephone contacts with the hospice nurse. The physician also has the crucial role of preparing the patient and family for the possibility that hospice might become an appropriate care choice and then recommending hospice care at the proper time. Every patient in hospice must have a physician involved in his or her care. The *hospice medical director,* who primarily acts as a consultant to the hospice team and to attending physicians, is less likely to have a direct relationship with the patient and family. Exceptions to this rule occur when the attending physician turns responsibility for the patient's care over to the medical director, when the patient has no other doctor, when the patient is in a hospice in-patient unit that the attending physician cannot visit, or when after-hours emergencies demand immediate medical intervention.

Rehabilitation therapists may become involved in hospice care when their services are needed to enhance the patient's comfort and physical functioning. These are the *physical* and *occupational therapist* and *speech/language pathologist* — each of whom helps patients recover from the debilitating effects of conditions such as strokes, paralysis, or amputations. Since their basic goal is rehabilitation — maximizing functioning and independence of chronically ill patients — their potential for achieving functional improvement in hospice is somewhat limited because the patients are dying. However, physical exercise programs, adaptive devices and equipment, and training for family caregivers may help the dying patient achieve the highest level of functioning possible for as long as possible. Speech pathologists also have suggestions for enhancing communication with patients who have lost the ability to speak, such as the use of communication sign boards.

The *pharmacist* is not likely to meet hospice patients, but provides valuable advice and recommendations to the hospice team about medications that could relieve the patient's symptoms, optimal dosages, interactions between various medications, and possibilities for easier and more effective drug administration. Hospice's relationship with the consulting pharmacist may also facilitate obtaining rare medications that aren't carried by the corner pharmacy or special preparations such as suppositories made from many of the medications used in hospice care.

The *consulting dietician* shares ideas and suggestions on how patients can cope with loss of appetite and still receive adequate nutrition, as well as on alternate forms of nutrition such as blenderized fruit drinks or nutritional supplements and special dietary concerns related to specific illnesses. Hospice dieticians have easy-to-use recipe books with simple ideas on how families can make meals more palatable for cancer patients. *Expressive arts therapists* — whether music, art or recreation — have a place in hospice care for patients who feel lonely, isolated, confused, tense, or otherwise in need of the enhanced quality of life that arts activities can offer. Expressive arts therapists in hospice are most often used with children, or in group in-patient settings. Formal *psychological care* — in addition to what is routinely provided by the social worker or chaplain — is not common in hospice. But some agencies have developed relationships with psychologists, psychiatrists, or family therapists to provide additional services such as consultation on difficult cases. The hospice team will let you know if any of these various ancillary services are available, or else they will be introduced on referral from your physician.

OTHER HOSPICE SERVICES

The full extent of other services offered by a hospice may be shaped by coverage under insurance benefits, and by what the physician and the hospice team recommend. Coverage is provided under the Medicare hospice benefit, under some private insurance plans — and by many hospices even when the patient does not have insurance coverage. The following items are routinely considered part of hospice: rented medical equipment such as hospital beds, wheelchairs, walkers, and commodes; oxygen equipment and tanks; basic medical supplies such as dressing changes, adult diapers, and gloves; egg crate mattresses and other assistive care devices; all prescription drugs needed to manage the terminal illness and the patient's comfort; and ambulance transfers when needed. Some of these items may come out of the hospice's free loan closet; others may have a small patient co-pay charge.

Another service provided by hospice is called *respite care,* which basically means a rest break for family caregivers, recognizing that the pressures of caring for a dying loved one can become very draining, physically and emotionally. Sometimes the hospice may place the patient on its in-patient unit or nursing home unit for up to five days, or else hospice staff or volunteers may fill shifts in the home, allowing the family to get out of the house for a few hours or a few days.

Under the Medicare hospice benefit, when medical crises arise in the patient's care, the hospice may provide more intensive *continuous nursing care* for eight to twenty-four hours per day in the home for short periods. Generally these crises are triggered by an acute symptom requiring the use of professional nursing staff to manage the patient's rapidly changing physical status. Medicare rules for continuous hospice care are complicated but can be explained by the hospice social worker. The rationale for continuous care is that while family caregivers are expected to play the major role in the ongoing care of their dying loved one, brief periods of continuous care can offer a safety net when caregiving demands become overwhelming for the family. A few days of continuous care by hospice may help bring the crisis back under control without the patient having to be hospitalized, and without the family throwing in the towel.

Patients and families considering hospice should also know that hospice does not include twenty-four-hour staffing in the home for extended periods of time. Home health aide or personal care aide visits may not always be as often or as long as the family might wish, depending on the hospice's policies and its perception of the patient's need. Medical treatments that the hospice believes to be curative in intent, such as experimental protocols or many kinds of chemotherapy, are not covered, nor are alternative treatments such as acupuncture or chiropractic. Hospice patients can and do pursue these treatments on their own, although they must pay for them out-of-pocket, unless they are covered under other parts of the person's health insurance policy.

🎝 Diane

Diane Reigel's mother was the first resident admitted to the House of the Dove Hospice Home, a seven-bed residential hospice program operated by St. Joseph's Hospital Hospice in Marshfield, Wisconsin, when it opened in 1989. Diane, one of five children, had been active in her mother's care, taking her to daily medical appointments to diagnose and then treat her cancer. Diane even traded off twelve-hour shifts with a brother to care for their mother, who was widowed and lived alone. "We took care of her for five weeks around the clock in her home. But I have a family of my own that I'm responsible for, with three young children," Diane explains.

When her mother had to be rehospitalized on St. Joseph's hospice inpatient unit, no longer able to walk, it became clear to the family that other arrangements were needed. Hospice staff suggested the House of the Dove. "She never regretted not going back home. She was here from the eighth of November, the day it opened, until February twenty-third," Diane says. "It was a big decision when we finally decided Mom should come here. There's a part of you that says you're giving up, but you're really not. You're taking care of yourself," she adds. Diane says she used the time visiting her mother at the House of the Dove to create memories, and to "make the best of right now. The house gave us the opportunity to have as much of a normal relationship as you can have with a dying mother. They took care of the hands-on care, so we could work with just the daily emotional stuff. My mother was relieved . . . because she was able to have a good rapport with her children, without being a burden."

Located in a former nuns' residence next door to St. Joseph's Hospital, House of the Dove had a few extra rooms on the second floor for use by family visitors. Another brother used to come from the southern part of the state to visit their mother and would stay overnight at the House. Greg Speltz, one of the facility's live-in "houseparents," relates that Diane's brother once told him the reason why he preferred to stay overnight at the House: "'My mother feels she is still my hostess when I stay here, and she's still taking care of me, because this is her home now. That's why I stay here.'"

CHAPTER FOUR

Additional Hospice Services

❧ Inpatient Care

For many families, their biggest questions about hospice center on the provision of inpatient care, the scope of this service, and its limitations. Most of the hospice services outlined in Chapter 3 are provided primarily or exclusively in the patient's home — which remains the major focus of hospice care. However, families often have doubts about their ability to care for the patient at home, to deal with the stresses of this responsibility, and to provide for the patient's safety and well-being. Even if they are willing to attempt it, they may still believe that it will eventually become impossible, or else they feel the need for some kind of escape clause should the responsibility become too great. When a family doubts its ability to care for the patient, hospice staff will often recommend just trying it, taking one day at a time, with the understanding that other approaches may become necessary later. For other patients, care at home is not an option — because they live alone, require constant supervision, or have no home to return to. What are the alternatives that hospice can offer to such patients and families?

An *inpatient hospice* is a health facility or unit in which arrangements have been made to provide an alternate setting for hospice care outside of the patient's home. Inpatient units may be separate wards or floors of a hospital or a nursing home, or else just a few beds at the end of the oncology unit. Other inpatient units are freestanding, located in a geographically distinct house or other building. Some American hospices have created elaborate inpatient units that are very special places — lovingly designed, attractive, and peaceful. Some of the features that characterize hospice inpatient units include variety in room design and larger rooms than in the typical health facility; family rooms with kitchenettes, privacy, and accommodations for staying overnight; lots of houseplants, artwork, and windows; and pleasant outdoor areas accessible to the residents. Generally hospice inpatient units offer flexible meal schedules, menu choices, and visiting hours and permission for children or even pets to visit the patient.

In fact, some families might take one look at the hospice's inpatient unit and declare that this is where they want their terminally ill loved one to be. Unfortunately, that's not always possible. Hospice inpatient units are often designed and staffed for short-term stays of only a few days or weeks, and generally can't be used indefinitely as the patient's long-term residence. Typical criteria for hospice inpatient admissions may include some of the following conditions: A newly enrolled hospice patient can be placed on the inpatient unit directly from the hospital for the first few days, to introduce the hospice program and bring pain under control, before returning home. Patients who are imminently dying may be placed on the unit for their last few days of life. Acute or emergency symptom management, defined broadly to recognize the interplay between physical, emotional, and social symptoms of terminal illness, may also necessitate placement on the unit. Family respite for rest and recuperation can be achieved by placing the patient on the unit for a few days. People with AIDS or with complicated medical care needs also have a greater need for inpatient care.

A new approach called *residential hospice care* has been developed in recent years for patients who don't fit into these categories. While residential care may look like inpatient care, there is an important distinction: Residential hospice care is designed for patients who do not need to be in a hospital, because their physical condition is relatively stable, yet they can't be in their own home or else don't have a home. It is intended for longer-term needs — months rather than days — but at a less intensive level of medical and nursing involvement. Most often the hospice residence is located in a converted private home with few of the institutional trappings of a hospital or nursing home. Some new freestanding hospice facilities have included both inpatient and residential levels of care under one roof. An outstanding example of this approach is a thirty-five-bed freestanding facility opened by Hospice of Dayton, Ohio, in 1990. Hospice residences such as Coming Home Hospice in San Francisco or House of the Dove Hospice Home in Marshfield, among others, are able to achieve a more truly homelike, informal atmosphere, with twenty-four-hour supervision for the residents provided collectively by personal-care aides or attendants. Usually, a registered nurse also visits the residence regularly and is available on-call for emergencies.

Other groups not affiliated with full-services hospice programs have also opened a number of residences or "hospice houses" around the country, primarily for people with AIDS. In fact, these "AIDS hospices" have made hospice more of a household word in some quarters than it was before the AIDS epidemic. However, the needs of terminally ill residents for twenty-four-hour supervision by personal care aides, for on-going case management and assessment by a registered nurse, in short for all of the coordinated services a hospice provides, make it imperative that the operators of these residences have close working relationships with a community hospice program. Otherwise, important physical-care needs may be neglected, eroding the resident's quality of life. The basic concept of a hospice house should be that a hospice home care team would come into the residence to provide hospice care the same as it does in patients' own homes.

Medicare and Medicaid hospice benefits recognize residential care to the extent of reimbursing the hospice at the same rate it receives for routine hospice care provided in a patient's home. However, room-and-board expenses — primarily for meals and rent — typically are not reimbursed under Medicare or insurance benefits. Therefore, the operators of hospice residences often must charge an additional room-and-board fee, on a sliding scale, to residents who are able to contribute to these costs.

Nursing home programs: in the absence of residential care options, hospices may make arrangements with nursing homes to provide a safe setting for hospice patients who can't be at home, using the resources of the hospice team to enhance the atmosphere and quality of life in the nursing home. Given the enormous number of elderly Americans already residing in nursing homes, and the fact that the nursing home is the usual solution to the medical and other needs of the chronically ill who can't be maintained safely in their own homes, some hospices have recognized that the nursing home *is* home for many potential clients. For those who have lived for years in a nursing home and have now become terminally ill, moving them out of the nursing home would be neither practical nor humane. Therefore, hospices are starting to work with nursing homes as a resource that already exists in their community.

However, the fact is that many people hold a negative perception of nursing homes as crowded, understaffed, or impersonal. There may be some truth to these perceptions, but more often nursing homes work very hard to give their residents the best care they can, within the constraints under which they operate. No one moves into a nursing home eagerly. The reason people are in nursing homes is that they didn't have other options. They were too old, too sick, too frail, or too confused to manage at home, and didn't have anyone willing and able to care for them. In a sense the nursing home is where our society dumps its most difficult medical and social problems, people with multiple chronic, long-term-care needs. Nursing homes are not given adequate financial resources to manage these cases, are heavily regulated and do not receive much respect for the work they do.

Some nursing homes have developed their own hospice programs, but the more common approach is for an existing community hospice to contract with the nursing home, spelling out how the hospice and the nursing home will each contribute to the care of the terminally ill nursing home resident. Under 1986 legislation extending Medicare hospice benefits to terminally ill, Medicaid-eligible nursing home residents, there now exists a reimbursement provision recognizing the nursing home as the patient's home for purposes of covering hospice care. Nursing home staff become the functional equivalent of the patient's family caregivers, and the hospice team enters into the nursing home the same as if it were the patient's own home. The hospice provides its basic services such as nurse, social worker, personal care aide, chaplain, volunteer, and medications that it would have provided in the patient's own home. The nursing home provides the same routine custodial services it would have provided anyway, such as meals, recreational activities, and bed linens. Nursing home staff provide twenty-four-hour supervision to the patient, but agree to call the hospice nurse when emergencies arise, while the hospice team directs and coordinates both sets of services under its plan of care for the patient.

The reimbursement for this arrangement is rather complicated. Either Medicaid or Medicare pays the hospice its customary daily rate for the "home care" services it provides to the nursing home resident. In lieu of the usual Medicaid reimbursement that would otherwise have been paid to the nursing home, Medicaid pays the hospice a second daily fee for additional "room and board" services, while the hospice then subcontracts with the nursing home for room and board. The hospice typically pays the facility a negotiated fee roughly the same as what the hospice receives for these services from Medicaid.

Terminally ill patients can qualify for such hospice-in-the-nursing-home services in one of two basic ways. They may already reside in the nursing home when they are diagnosed as being terminally ill, with six months or less to live, and then opt to receive hospice care. Otherwise, they may be patients of a community hospice who are no longer able to remain in their own homes and now must be placed in a substitute home setting, so they enter a nursing home with which the hospice contracts. In either case, the success of this collaboration depends on the ability of the hospice and nursing home to devise and execute a functional working agreement clearly specifying their corresponding tasks and responsibilities. If it is done well, the terminally ill patient should be receiving every kind of hospice support he or she would have received at home, had it been possible to remain at home, plus a more intensive level of hands-on care and supervision than other residents of the same nursing home are likely to get. The hospice also provides bereavement support to families after the patient's death.

Finally, an approach tried in a few localities is the *hospice day care program,* a concept borrowed from geriatric adult day health care centers. Hospice patients continue to live in their own homes, but are transported to the hospice day care center one or more days a week during business hours, for group activities and support. This approach is especially helpful for patients whose caregivers must work during the day, since the caregiver can go to work while the patient receives adequate supervision during working hours.

LIMITATIONS TO INPATIENT CARE

The limitations placed on hospice inpatient care can be frustrating for some families, but it may be helpful to keep in mind a few basic facts about the contemporary American health care system within which hospices, too, must operate. Hospital care in America, with its panoply of high-tech equipment and highly trained specialists, has become very expensive, running up to a thousand dollars a day. Given the ever more complicated rules and limitations of Medicare and insurance companies aimed at containing hospital costs, hospitals today find themselves financially obligated to make their patients' stays as brief as possible. Patients need a very good medical reason, usually related to the need for highly technical treatments, in order to justify remaining hospitalized overnight — even when they are dying. Nursing homes are often the next stop for seriously ill patients who must leave the hospital, but today even nursing homes need to demon-strate that their patients have a genuine need for nursing care that justifies a continued stay in the facility. Home health agencies face similar pressures to document that the patients they serve at home are physically confined to the home and in need of professional rehabilitative services.

This is the milieu in which hospices operate, and the poli-cies of Medicare and insurance companies essentially dictate that hospice patients who are placed on inpatient units should also have genuine, specific medical reasons for being there. As a result, hospice inpatient units may only be able to keep pa-tients on the unit for several days or a couple of weeks, while specific medical problems such as pain are stabilized, but not for prolonged periods of maintenance care that could be sup-plied equally well at home. Inpatient care is also referred to as acute care, and is provided on hospice units that are required to meet many of the same regulations as hospitals.

The alternative to acute care is to provide hospice within residential facilities or nursing homes, where lower levels of professional staffing and less intensive care and equipment help keep costs down, which in turn means that longer stays are possible. However, because of the costs of building or ac-quiring a residence and the lack of insurance reimbursement to cover ongoing room and board expenses for hospice resi-dences, most hospices are not able to offer this option. Another option is the nursing home, but for many patients and families, this will seem like an inadequate solution. There may also be regulations and procedures required of the nurs-ing home, or environmental factors within the facility, that are not conducive to optimal hospice care. Families with ques-tions about these issues should call their local hospice to clarify what care options are open to them. But they should also be aware that hospice care is generally designed to be provided in the home and to supplement the family's caregiving responsibilities — not to replace the family.

🦜 Hospice Bereavement Services

One final type of service provided by hospices is designed to address the grief support needs of family caregivers *after* the patient dies. The hospice philosophy recognizes the powerful emotional and physical changes experienced following the death of a loved one, and hospices continue serving family members for a year or more after the patient's death. Bereavement services provided by hospices vary considerably from agency to agency. Generally they are available to the primary family caregiver of hospice patients, and often to other family members of friends who are also dealing with the loss. Many hospices also offer some or all of their bereavement services to the larger community, for people who have experienced other losses, such as a sudden death, an illness in which hospice did not participate, or the death of a relative receiving care in a distant community.

The basic goals of hospice bereavement services for the survivors of hospice patients include the following: (1) Hospice tries to normalize the grief experience by reminding survivors that what they are experiencing is perfectly nor-mal, even though they may feel that they are going crazy. (2) Hospice provides education about the grief process and information about how to cope with it. Hospice grief counselors emphasize that this is a long and difficult process, and remind clients to get adequate rest, relaxation, exercise, and nutrition in the meantime. (3) Hospice offers survivors information about issues they may not have had to consider while the patient was alive, such as driving a car, paying bills and taxes, or doing routine home maintenance. (4) Hospice encourages survivors to tell their story and to talk about their loss, over and over again if necessary, until it is talked through. (5) Hospice offers emotional support, companionship, and understanding to help mitigate some of the worst pangs of grief, supporting the client's hopes that this experience can be survived and eventually resolved. (6) If the individual's grief experience is particularly troubling, protracted, or delayed, hospice may provide additional resources and referrals for more intensive professional help.

Generally hospices place their emphasis on routine support for the majority of bereaved clients who are experiencing normal grief reactions, although they also try to identify and respond to the smaller number who may be at risk for more serious problems. While most people are able to work through their own grief without outside help, hospice bereavement professionals believe they can help make this process a little easier to manage, and perhaps even a little shorter in duration, by offering emotional support to survivors. A much smaller number of the bereaved need extra attention and more structured professional guidance through their grief.

It is common for hospice staff and volunteers to attend their patients' wakes, funeral home visitations, funeral services, or the scattering of cremated ashes, if invited by the family. Generally the patient's primary nurse and social worker will visit the family at least one more time shortly after the patient's death. They, too, may be grieving the loss, and will want to say good-bye to the family so they can move on to new cases. They may still be in touch occasionally, but at this point they introduce a new team of bereavement caregivers who have special grief counseling skills. The hospice bereavement team typically includes a bereavement coordinator, one or more professionally trained grief counselors and

support group facilitators, and bereavement volunteers —
generally people who have experienced and worked through
significant losses in their own lives.

Initiation of hospice bereavement services may be delayed for a month or more after the death, until the acute
shock experienced by the bereaved starts to wear off. Among
its other services the hospice may offer a schedule of *phone
calls to grieving family members* at regular intervals: one month,
three months, and six months after the death. Alternatively or
in addition, there may be *monthly mailings* announcing the
availability of hospice bereavement services, with brief informational pamphlets about grief and the bereavement process,
bereavement newsletters, or anniversary cards. Families may
be offered home visits by the *bereavement volunteer,* whose primary responsibility is to encourage the survivor to talk about
the loss and perhaps get out of the house and go to a restaurant for lunch. There may also be *formalized grief counseling* at
the hospice office, for a limited number of sessions, as well
as referrals to other mental health professionals for more intensive counseling. However, while routine phone calls or
mailings will be made to every family, unless the family
specifically asks not to receive them, face-to-face services usually are only utilized if the family wants them. Offers of services may be made several times; if they aren't wanted
immediately, they may be more useful a few months down
the road.

Hospices also offer a variety of group settings for bereavement support, in one of three main types. *Educational groups*
provide important information on grief and coping, with a specific curriculum for a limited number of sessions, perhaps six to
eight weeks. Such groups might also teach personal finances,
cooking for one, traveling alone, and coping with the holidays.
Mutual support/self help groups are the traditional support group

model in which people with similar problems get together to talk about their feelings, usually with the guidance of a professional facilitator. Often these groups are targeted at a specific population: widows and widowers, survivors of AIDS patients, minor children who have experienced a significant loss, or grieving parents. It's not uncommon for the participants in such groups to form close friendships and continue getting together socially after the formal, facilitated group has concluded. *Hospice social events* may combine festivities, food, and drink with a safe, pleasant environment to meet and talk with other survivors and with familiar hospice staff. Sometimes two or more of these basic group formats or approaches may be combined in one meeting.

Two final bereavement services that may be offered by a hospice are a *lending library* of books and videos on grief-related topics, for anyone seeking additional information and guidance, and *memorial services* or remembrance rituals. Some hospices put on their own memorial service, once or twice a year, for the families of patients who have died in recent months. These services tend to be ecumenical and informal, offering families an opportunity to publicly acknowledge the loss of a loved one. Other such rituals include "Tree of Life" celebrations now held annually in many communities, in which lights are placed on a publicly displayed Christmas tree in honor of people who have died. This celebration is usually open to the entire community, not just the survivors of hospice patients. Call your local hospice for more information on which of these various bereavement services — or others — are offered, and whether they are available to the wider community or only to survivors of that hospice's patients. Most of these services, with the possible exception of professional grief counseling sessions, are offered without charge or at minimal cost.

Betty V.

Betty Vaughn, who lost her husband, Chuck, four months ago, at home and under the care of HospiceCare in Madison, Wisconsin, says, "Hospice couldn't have been more full of empathy and caring, and they did just exactly what needed to be done but without being intrusive. I am so grateful to them. But you get kind of numb. I have had to reread the sympathy notes again because I didn't take it all in at first. You know, you're talking about someone you spent forty years of your life with, and you get numb and tune out. I'm gradually returning to some of my former activities, and now I'm trying to pick up the pieces again. But there's a void there," says Betty.

"Everything I've read about grief says that there are stages of recovery. I have a friend who calls me, who lost his wife; we were close couples. He'll say, 'Well, what stage of grief are you in now?' And I'll have to say, 'I don't know exactly, but for instance, I am a little better than I was,'" she relates. "I think you gradually reach out, as you can handle it. But there are little down spots all the time. I can be doing quite well and think, oh, isn't this a wonderful day, and I have a reason to get up. And then something will come along and pull me down again, like someone will call on the phone and ask for my husband. Usually it's a salesperson, and it's awfully hard for me to say he can't come to the phone. Holidays are especially hard. I have a bad memory for Christmas at the moment, but I'll get over that," she adds.

"One book I read says widowhood is the last stage of life. You feel so mortal, you see. . . . I've had to say to myself: 'Are you feeling sorry for yourself a bit?' I think in recovering you have to think about that a little, figuring out when the horrible grief and the empty spot are handled, and when you get into just feeling sorry for yourself," she explains. "I've come out of this wanting to seize the moment — treasuring every day that I feel so healthy and energetic and want to do things. You know in the long picture we are such a short time on this planet. Some things just don't bother me like they used to — that's one of the pluses. I'm also a better person at feeling empathy for someone else who has a life-threatening illness, and at writing sympathy notes, which used to be so tough for me," she says.

Betty now gives a lot attention to Chuck's favorite cat, an arthritic Siamese. "I'm doing everything possible to keep her in good health, because my husband loved her so, and it's like a little part of him." She's also exploring legacies, such as having a brick engraved with his name placed in the garden walkway of the local botanical garden, or helping the Madison hospice to expand its memorial giving program. "I don't mean it to be a morbid thing about someone that's gone, but I don't want to forget him," she says. "I'm trying to pull up the good memories. I find myself talking about something he did, and I like that. I want to keep him alive, for friends and relatives as well as for myself."

CHAPTER FIVE

The Referral Process: Making the First Call

*Families who won't let us begin working with them until the very
end of the illness, until the patient is close to death, almost
without exception will say, "Gosh, I wish we had let
you start working with us earlier."*
— J. Mark Springer,
chaplain, Hospice of Louisville, Kentucky

What happens when you call hospice? Whom do you call, and
when? In practice it is usually a simpler process than one
might think, because hospices try to make it easy for people
who have taken that important first step and picked up the
telephone. Requests for hospice services can come from many
sources: potential clients, their relatives, friends, neighbors,
roommates, employers, or ministers — in short from anyone
who is concerned about and involved in the patient's life and
care. Hospice referrals also come from physicians, clinic
nurses, hospital social workers or discharge planners, home
health agencies, nursing homes, health maintenance organizations, or insurance company case managers.

Patients, their families, and friends may have read about
hospice in newspapers or magazines, or they may have heard

about it on radio or television. By now, so many Americans already have experience with hospice care for a dying loved one that it's possible a friend or relative can offer a personal testimonial. Hospice brochures can be obtained in doctors' offices or medical resource libraries, or from groups like the American Cancer Society, the National Consumers League, or the Government Printing Office (for Medicare beneficiaries). In most communities you can simply open the telephone directory yellow pages to "hospice" and find the numbers of local hospice providers.

Once the call has been made to hospice, what happens next depends on the patient's needs and on the hospice's policies. Some hospices will offer to send callers written information about their services and make arrangements to talk again in a few days. Others will immediately transfer the call to their intake department, where trained professionals can start gathering essential information and explaining hospice procedures. It should not be upsetting if the person who answers the hospice's telephone asks to take the caller's name and number to have someone return the call later. The person who is best equipped to handle intake calls may not always be available at the moment a potential client decides to call hospice. If someone other than the patient or immediate family member has placed the initial call on the patient's behalf, the hospice may ask them to get the patient's permission before the case can proceed. It would be awkward for the hospice to contact a patient who is not expecting or desiring such a call.

It may take several phone calls to amass enough information to initiate hospice services. If the patient's needs are urgent, the hospice may try to expedite the intake process, but it's probably not realistic to expect the first call to hospice to result in same-day or weekend admission. Early in this process, hospice representatives will also ask for permission to talk to the attending physician about the case, if the physician isn't already involved.

The referral process also explores what the patient knows about his or her prognosis, other medical concerns, the patient's family and living situation, and expectations for care. These questions can sometimes raise painful issues for the family, but it is important that everyone be clear from the outset what enrollment in hospice means, so that the patient, family, and doctor can all give free and informed consent to hospice care. Issues such as treatment options and the patient's wishes regarding heroic measures such as resuscitation also need to be spelled out if the hospice is to respect and promote the patient's wishes.

Some of these questions can't be fully answered at first because of the family's stress and lack of knowledge about hospice and other options. There is only so much information that can be taken in all at once, and the stress families are under affects their comprehension. The longer-term issues will be revisited by hospice staff during subsequent visits, and questions that are just too painful for families to discuss in the beginning may be postponed until their anxiety level has been reduced. Hospice will also ask about health insurance policies and coverage and — if there is none — whether the patient and family might be able to contribute financially to the costs of their care. However, hospice programs customarily do not turn away a patient in need because of an inability to pay.

At some point, usually within one or a few days of the first phone call to hospice, the admission process shifts from the telephone to an in-person visit in the patient's home or hospital room, usually by the intake specialist or by the nurse who will be assuming primary case management responsibil-

ity for the patient's care. This intake visit may include an assessment of the patient's physical condition and vital signs by
the nurse, a discussion of the roles family and friends can play
in the patient's care, and a review of hospice policies and services. Then, if everyone agrees, the patient may be asked to
read and sign the hospice informed consent form. If the patient is not ready to sign, or is not sure, hospice staff can leave
the written information in the home and give the patient a
chance to think it over. Some hospices now also have "pre-
hospice" programs through which they can offer limited
counseling, advice, and other services to patients who aren't
yet ready or able to commit to the full hospice approach.

An example of such pre-hospice services is Program
Care, a service of Hospice of Central Kentucky in Elizabethtown, designed for people with cancer, whether their status is newly diagnosed, under active treatment, or terminal.
"We try to serve as a hospice team in limited ways," says
Program Care coordinator Jan Swope. Some clients may eventually transfer over to formal hospice services, but for those
who don't, Program Care provides emotional support, information, encouragement for self-education, and referrals to
other community resources. "They have lots of needs, some
similar to hospice, some not," Swope says. "When one hears a
diagnosis of cancer, it's pretty scary. People's lives just tem-
porarily seem to come unraveled." Although Program Care
was originally conceived in part as a way to acquaint cancer
patients with the hospice program, so that they might transfer
to hospice when their disease reaches the terminal phase, in
reality this doesn't often happen. "Part of our goal is to help
folks newly diagnosed with cancer to go on and live as long as
possible," Swope says.

Hospice services officially commence when the patient
signs the consent form. Once the patient is enrolled, then the

hospice team shifts into high gear. The next nursing and social work visits are planned. Delivery of needed equipment is arranged. Medication schedules and supplies are checked. Patients and families are asked if they want other services, for instance, a hospice volunteer or chaplain. And the whole hospice approach gradually unfolds, with the hospice team doing everything possible to make the patient and family's journey smoother and easier. In fact, for many patients and families, what happens once hospice care starts will be easier and more straightforward than what preceded it. The harder parts are choosing the hospice alternative and making that first call.

🦋 *The Physician's Role in Hospice Referrals*

Although the decision to enroll in hospice ultimately lies with the patient and family, much of the responsibility for how this process unfolds lies with the patient's doctor. In fact, research done at the University of Louisville in the mid-1980s describes the doctor's role in introducing hospice to patients as the crucial factor in the family's hospice decision. Researchers in the university's Urban Studies Center conducted a large-scale study of the decision-making process leading up to enrollment in hospice by interviewing patients, families, doctors, and other health professionals. While their research is now several years old, it still offers one of the best glimpses into what really happens during the painful and difficult process of deciding to receive hospice care.

This research showed that while three-fourths of Kentucky families experiencing the death of a family member to cancer in 1985 had heard of hospice, they were unlikely to act on knowledge about hospice received prior to the family member's illness. Only when information on hospice was given to them when it was relevant to their immediate situation was this information likely to be used. "General knowledge about hospice is not enough; only when information is offered *after* the family has learned the terminal nature of the disease is that information influential. Only when someone specifically suggests that hospice might be appropriate for them, do people consider hospice," the researchers state. The relevant information at the relevant time was most likely to be given by a health professional, usually the attending physician. Researchers also discovered that if the physician introduced or recommended hospice care at the appropriate time, then families were likely to use the service, but if the physician did not, then families were not likely to receive hospice care. Unfortunately, researchers found, "the medical community does not routinely offer this information to patients and families." Only half of surveyed physicians introduced the hospice option to their terminally ill patients.

The person making the decision to receive hospice care was usually the family caregiver closest to the patient, typically a spouse, parent, or child, and the decision was usually made with the involvement of few other people. The patient's role in the decision-making process was often limited, no doubt because of the effects of the illness and medications. It also makes sense that the person most active in providing the patient's care, coordinating treatment schedules and doctor's visits, and arranging for a host of other needs, would also be the one to make the decision about hospice care, based on whether or not hospice seemed likely to make the caregiving role easier to handle.

When a person has been diagnosed with cancer, family members and health professional both will try to be as encouraging and hopeful as possible. The last thing patients and families who are mobilizing their strength to fight the disease want to hear about is the hospice option for terminal care, awaiting them should treatment fail. Thus, their general knowledge about hospice is often simply not relevant or useful until someone in a position of authority, such as the doctor, draws its connection to their circumstances and to the fact that the disease has apparently reached the terminal stage. They may need to be told that this is the time to seek the help that hospice can provide.

The transition to hospice is often described as shifting gears or changing the direction of care. An approach of trying to overcome the illness medically is replaced by the hospice approach of palliative, or comfort, care. The medical facts may make this decision obvious: either no promising treatments are available, or else available treatments have prohibitively severe side effects. Other times the hospice decision may be based on trade-offs, a comparison of the personal costs and benefits of continued treatment versus palliative care. Most often patients depend on the doctor to tell them when the time is right for hospice. How does this actually work? For oncologists, it is known as "the conversation" — an intimate discussion that takes place in the privacy of the doctor's office, or else at the hospital bedside, often with family members present. Sometimes it is not a single conversation, but instead a process that goes on over time, preparing the patient emotionally for the transition to hospice.

"The hospice decision really is a hurdle for some patients," says William Medina, M.D., a Lexington, Kentucky, oncologist. "They really do change gears at that point, so it's important that it's done properly. It's a difficult issue, and a lot of things go into it. We almost never reach a point in cancer where there's absolutely nothing else we can do" to fight the disease, he explains. "I think it's also fair to say that hospice isn't for everybody. Some people just either don't need it all, even though they're dying, or else because of their personality it's just not going to be a positive experience for them." A minority of Medina's patients say they want to fight the disease "to the bitter end. There are some people who I wish wouldn't. I may try to talk them out of it, if side effects are likely to be prohibitive, compared with potential benefits. But there, again, you have to be careful how you phrase it." Introducing the hospice option "can be a painful conversation. I think you have to slide into it, work your way into it. I usually talk about it from the point of view of options," Medina explains. "It's important, because you're making a statement about their future: 'This doesn't mean we're giving up on you. We're just going to change tactics here.'"

"Not many patients come in and say, 'I want to get hooked up with hospice,'" explains Peter Kohler, M.D., a Madison, Wisconsin, oncologist. "It's usually from our end that we bring up the idea of hospice. Once you use that word 'hospice,' the connotation it gives is: That's it. Even though they know they have a terminal disease, even though those words have been there, it's like hospice is the coup de grace. Many of these people, once they get hooked up with the organization, are some of its biggest praisers. Not uncommonly we'll just say to patients, 'Why don't you talk to hospice? You're not buying anything, just talk to them, hear what they have to say, see what they can do, and if you think it might help, go with it,'" Kohler relates. "Usually you know these people as a physician. For the most part you've seen them at the time they were diagnosed, and you go with them through the course of their disease. You have a certain rapport established. So when it gets to that point it becomes a relatively easy conversation, in the sense that they know you're trying to give them the best care possible. It becomes more difficult when I get thrown into a situation where practically the first word out of my mouth is hospice."

Often, Kohler says, cancer patients will remain at a certain plateau with their disease, "and then finally they hit the edge and start to slide. Usually it's over pain control issues, or not being able to function up to par, and the need to have some support, somebody coming out to the house," he explains. "If I get a sense in the course of an office visit that things are not going well at home, and we need to get somebody in, I'll come right out and say it: 'I think it would be a wise idea for you to start thinking about an organization like hospice that can come out and start helping you make decisions about your medicines, and those kinds of things.'"

But there are other patients, says Kohler's office nurse, Sue Frankewicz, "who over the course of their therapy come to realize by themselves that the journey they are on is not where they wanted to be. They come to realize that they are dying. A fair number initiate their own consults with hospice. Others will give us subtle hints in their comments: 'Well, I've got my will done, I've got my things wrapped up. I know who I'm leaving my money to.' And those are signals that people recognize that their life is nearing an end," Frankewicz suggests.

"Patients can initiate a hospice referral themselves," says a Madison oncologist, Edward Prendergast, M.D. "I usually say, wonderful! They may have gotten ahead of me in the game." Sometimes the treatment picture may not look very good, but the patient and doctor are each looking to the other for some cue that it's time to start talking about different directions. Patients may need help from an office nurse or hospital social worker to initiate a discussion with doctors who are uncomfortable making hospice referrals. "A lot of times doctors are waiting for a signal from the family," says Joseph Ousley,

M.D., medical director of St. Joseph's Hospital Hospice in Marshfield, Wisconsin. "They have to maintain their traditional mode of action until they get some signal from the family or patient that it's okay to stop trying so hard."

"There are very few people who unilaterally stop treatments which are working, in my experience," Kohler adds. "It's usually obvious to them and obvious to us that whatever we're doing, the balance isn't there, it's costing too much. There's an old adage that if it was working you'd be feeling better, and if you're not feeling better it usually tells us it's not working." Chemotherapy can make patients feel rotten at times, he explains, "but there should also be points where you're back up to your baseline condition or better." Other cancer patients say, "I'm gonna lick it! I want all the chemotherapy that you've got,'" Kohler relates. That can be difficult for the physician, "because there's a point where you have more drugs than patient," he adds. "They have to come to a realization of what the situation is. Then hospice becomes an integral part of helping them carry out what they've realized. It's part of the process that perhaps the difficulties people have in dealing with hospice are really just a reflection of their difficulty in dealing with the whole picture of their terminal diagnosis," Kohler says.

"I saw a man just a few hours ago and had to decide whether to talk to him about hospice," says William Hocking, M.D., head of the oncology department at the Marshfield Clinic. "He's been ill for about three years with a carcinoid tumor that's generally a fairly slowly progressing tumor. And that's been his course, but he's now reached a point where he doesn't want further active treatments or resuscitation. But at the same time, he has not wanted to think of himself as dying. I decided it was appropriate to talk to him and his wife about hospice today. His wife was quite enthusiastic, and he was very resistant because he felt I was saying he's going to die. And I told him: 'Going into the hospice program itself will have no impact on your life span. The purpose of going into the hospice is to make the duration of your life a higher quality than it would be otherwise.' After I said that he agreed to meet with the hospice nurse," Hocking says.

"The thing I want people to understand is that hospice is an adjunct," says David Zoeller, M.D., an Elizabethtown, Kentucky, family practitioner. "It doesn't replace any of your doctors," he says. "I try to point out: 'You have a terminal illness. The odds are not very good. You can be hopeful, but let's also be realistic. You may have certain things you want to get done. You don't have that much time left, probably. We can hope, in the time you've got left, to make the quality as good as it can be.' "

🌿 Linda

Linda Welch's mother was diagnosed with cancer in 1988. Linda lives in Louisville, Kentucky, but her parents were in rural Hardin Country, so they came into Louisville by bus for the radiation treatments. Later her mother was hospitalized for fluid buildup in her lungs, "and at that point the doctor told us we needed to talk to someone from hospice. From the outset we all had a good rapport with the people who came out from hospice. But it was most important that Mother had a good rapport with them, and she did seem to. I don't think we could have gotten through it without hospice," she adds.

"Momma and I had been at odds and had a very stressed relationship for many years," Linda reveals. "I wanted to do something — you know how you always want to . . . wipe the slate clean. But it was so hard to do that with Momma. So I contacted Mary, the hospice social worker. I told her that I knew Mother's needs came first, but if there was a way, I'd like to get some things squared away with Mother. I had not known that Mother had pretty much told her the same thing. So with Mary's help we actually did sit down together, but it was so late in her illness that Mother didn't have the strength — the breath in her — really to talk that much. We only had the opportunity for one or two sessions with Mary."

Linda recalls that on the day before her mother died, "the social worker took me out of the hospital room and said, 'You know, there are things that your mother has wanted to say, and now she doesn't have the breath to do it. But if you're willing, I know the issues that your mother has wanted to deal with. There's nothing you can say to your mother right now that's going to hurt her. She's in a different place. If there's something you really want to say, don't worry about hurting her feelings. She can take whatever you have to say.' So we went in and we talked and it was, I guess, one of the best things that I've ever been able to do. Mother couldn't really talk, but she took her (oxygen) mask off, and she said, 'I love you,' with all the breath that she had in her, and put her mask back on. And I thought, jeez, in all my years my mother has never said that to me. So that was hard, but it was important. I don't think I would have had the courage to do that if I hadn't had the support I got from the people here at hospice," Linda says. Since her mother's death, the hospice has continued to help Linda with one-on-one grief counseling and grief support groups, as she struggles with her loss.

CHAPTER SIX

Hospice Providers, Coverage, and Access Issues

> *Hospice exists in the hope and belief that, through appropriate care
> and the promotion of a caring community sensitive to their needs,
> patients and families may be free to attain a degree of mental and
> spiritual preparation for death that is satisfying to them.*
> — *"Standards for a Hospice Program of Care,"*
> *developed by the National Hospice Organization*

Models of Hospice Programs

While the hospice movement in this country is barely nineteen years old, it has grown dramatically to more than sixteen hundred operational hospices located in every state and
covering all but the most rural or isolated parts of the country. Most hospice programs are either separate entities or else
affiliated with another independent health care organization,
such as a hospital. While hospices may voluntarily participate as members of state and national trade associations
such as the National Hospice Organization or the Hospice
Association of America, they are not chapters or offices of a
nationwide corporate entity. In other words, these national

associations have no direct control over the operation of your neighborhood hospice. As a result, there will be significant variations among hospices in the extent of services they provide, in eligibility criteria, in the nature and organization of inpatient services (if any), in whether they qualify for hospice benefits paid by Medicare, Medicaid, or private insurance plans, and in whether and how they serve children, people with AIDS, patients living alone, or others with special needs.

Roughly three-fourths of U.S. hospices qualify for Medicare or Medicaid reimbursement and can provide the federally defined hospice benefits available to beneficiaries of those programs. Certain health maintenance organizations or insurance companies may contract with a limited number of hospices or may even have in-house hospice programs for their own beneficiaries only. Veterans Affairs Medical Centers increasingly will be offering hospice services to eligible veterans. Outlined below are some of the key questions that consumers can ask their local hospice to help sort out the variations that may be relevant to their situation. In all cases, the emphasis of hospice should be on caring humanely and expertly for people who have terminal or life-threatening illnesses, and on identifying and meeting their personal needs for comfort, support, and dignity in a nonjudgmental way. However, this basic approach has been adapted and revised to local needs, local circumstances, and available resources within each community.

Hospices can be divided into a few basic categories that may influence the range of services they provide. *Community-based* hospices are independent, nonprofit corporations governed by a community board of directors in order to meet the needs of the dying in the community. The advantage of the community-based hospice is that it has no other mission and no higher priority than caring for the dying; the disadvantage is that such programs may not enjoy the financial stability and support that comes from being part of a larger organization.

Home health agency–based hospices are part of home care agencies such as Visiting Nurses Associations or Public Health Nursing Departments. Within such agencies the hospice may be a separate and distinct program, or it may be closely integrated into the larger agency's home care staffing and services. Home health agencies are generally considered functionally the type of health care provider closest to hospice, but there are some crucial differences between typical home health agency services and true hospice care. Home health agency staff, no matter how skilled, do not have hospice's specialization in terminal care. Also, home health care reimbursement customarily does not permit the time or the intensity of care that is provided by the hospice nurse, nor does it incorporate the full range of services provided by a hospice, including, for example, bereavement support for surviving family members.

Hospital–based hospices are administratively part of a hospital corporation. They may provide some or all of their services in the patient's home, but often the services are closely integrated with the parent facility and are located on or near the oncology unit. *Nursing home–based* hospices are similar to hospital-based ones in the sense that their affiliation with the larger facility doesn't always indicate the focus of their services. A corner or wing of the nursing home may be turned into a specialized hospice unit, or else the nursing home–based hospice program may provide its services in patients' homes, or both. Health facility–based hospices can easily draw upon the various ancillary services of the larger facility, but the needs of a small hospice department sometimes get lost in a large institution that places too much emphasis on the bottom line.

In a few communities *coalition-model* hospices work cooperatively with a number of other local providers, such as home health agencies, in order to offer a range of hospice services. The coalition hospice doesn't provide professional services directly but instead coordinates and facilitates nursing and other care provided by other agencies. Such hospices do not qualify for reimbursement, and they may run into problems when they can't directly control the patient care provided by the other agencies.

Volunteer-intensive hospices also belong to one of the other categories or models. Regardless of their organizational affiliation, however, these tend to be small, usually rural agencies providing most or all of their services through the use of volunteers, sometimes even in professional or administrative capacities. They may not have the resources to provide the full range of hospice services, but the special caring and spirit that comes from the work of volunteers is hard to beat. In small or isolated communities the volunteer hospice may be the only option possible.

Freestanding hospice is a term that usually refers to a hospice inpatient unit which has been set up in a geographically distinct building. Freestanding hospice units have more control over the atmosphere and the procedures of inpatient care than do hospice units located in hospitals or nursing homes, but they may not be as cost-effective. *Residential* hospices, also known as hospice houses, in contrast to inpatient units, aim to provide longer-term, substitute homelike settings of care for patients who cannot be cared for in their own homes. Staffing and intensity of services are comparable to a board-and-care home or other type of licensed residential facility.

Often a residential hospice program will be operated by a home care hospice, or else by an independent agency that contracts with a community hospice for professional services needed by its residents.

A small number of hospices are also based within health maintenance organizations, such as the Kaiser Permanente health plan in California, or Group Health Cooperative of Puget Sound in Washington, or in other health care–related organizations such as Veterans' Affairs Medical Centers. Kaiser, the nation's largest HMO, offers hospice care as a benefit in many of its regions, and often has full-service hospice teams based in its medical centers.

A few American hospices are *proprietary*, or privately owned, profit-making enterprises. The largest of these, VITAS Innovative Hospice Care (formerly called Hospice Care, Inc., of Delaware), with main offices in Miami, operates hospice programs in the states of Florida, Texas, and Illinois. Its ability to turn a financial profit on hospice care is based in part on its aggressive marketing outreach to attract new patients, and on its large size and resulting operational economies of scale — since a single central administration can provide management support and services for a large number of professional staff serving many patients. To some in the American hospice movement, a proprietary hospice seems somehow contrary to hospice's idealistic tradition, as does the aggressive marketing of hospice services. However, there is no evidence that proprietary hospices are less expert or dedicated in the care they provide, or that their services are less satisfactory to patients and families.

These, then, are the basic models of hospice in terms of their internal organization and control. The differences between these hospice models or types generally is less important than their similarities as hospices. Another way of classifying hospices is in terms of the external standards and regulations they meet. Such external standards come in three basic forms: licensure, certification, and accreditation.

Licensure is defined by state statutes, typically under the consumer protection code. The rationale for licensure is that a consumer using a state-licensed hospice should be assured that this hospice meets minimum requirements for a hospice program, as defined by state regulations. Slightly more than half of the states now have hospice licensure laws in effect, and several others are in the process of implementing them. In some states there may be different levels or categories of hospice licensure, for example, full-service versus volunteer. Some hospice programs may also obtain a license in another state-defined category of health service or facility, such as home health agency, skilled nursing facility, or specialized hospital. While such crossovers may be confusing to the consumer, they mostly reflect the hospice's need to meet *some* state standards or to qualify for health insurance reimbursement. Which category of licensure a hospice possesses is less important to the consumer than whether the hospice meets all applicable state standards. The state Department of Health or Consumer Affairs can often help sort out consumers' questions about hospice licensure.

Certification for hospices means that they have been examined by government surveyors and found to meet the minimum requirements for participation in Medicare. Thus they are able to provide hospice services and be paid for such services under Medicare. If your state has a Medicaid hospice benefit (and more than half do), then certified hospices will also qualify to provide this benefit. Certification is important to the consumer because it means the hospice can access valuable benefits paid by Medicare or Medicaid, and thus offer a greater range of services such as medical equipment, supplies, and medications free or nearly free to covered patients. Roughly three-quarters of American hospices today qualify for the Medicare program, and these generally tend to be larger programs with full-time paid staff. A hospice program that is not certified can still provide hospice services, but will not be paid by Medicare.

The third category of standards for hospices to meet is called *accreditation*. As with accreditation of colleges and universities, an accredited hospice has been found to meet a higher standard of quality by an independent, nongovernmental monitoring body. Generally accreditation is a voluntary process and therefore should demonstrate a hospice's commitment to being a high-quality enterprise. So it is always a positive sign for consumers. Until recently the Joint Commission on Accreditation of Healthcare Organizations, the national organization that accredits hospitals, also offered a program to accredit hospices. A few hospices today may still carry an unexpired "seal of approval" from the Joint Commission. Unfortunately, the Joint Commission decided in 1990 to terminate its respected hospice accreditation program for financial reasons and because of a lack of participation by hospices.

This decision has created a quandary for those hospices that are truly committed to being the very best they can be, and who want a recognized way to demonstrate that commitment. The Community Health Accreditation Program, a subsidiary of the National League for Nursing, began accrediting hospices in 1989, but its program for hospices is so new that few have yet participated. At least one state hospice organization, in Oregon, also accredits hospices according to standards it has developed. As with licensure, hospices may find it useful to be accredited and reviewed in other health provider categories, such as health facility or home health agency.

When considering a potential provider of hospice care, it is worth asking whether that hospice is licensed, certified, or accredited, but you must also ask which of these standards actually apply in your state, and under what conditions. At the same time, it should be remembered that these standards are designed to be applied broadly, for a large number of agencies across a state or across the country. Thus they may not always recognize the unique advantages and disadvantages of an individual hospice program. Whether or not a hospice is flexible enough to tailor a plan of care to a patient's unique circumstances and then deliver that care competently and reliably is just as important as external quality standards. It is up to the consumer to ask informed questions of the hospice provider before services are initiated.

There is another approach that might be encountered in exploring options for people with life-threatening illnesses, from agencies that claim their services are "just like hospice" or "just as good as hospice" or "hospice-like." Obviously many health care organizations were providing care for dying patients long before hospice came on the scene, and many continue to provide high quality care, using a variety of methods in a variety of settings for people with terminal or life-threatening illnesses. There may be valid reasons why a health care organization would not offer true hospice services, even though it takes care of people with life-threatening illnesses. It may be that the agency's clients don't want the hospice approach, or that the agency's services already meet their needs. There may also be structural or administrative or regulatory barriers preventing development of a true hospice program.

In fact, other providers of terminal care in a community may be as good as the hospice, offering high-quality care to dying patients. There may be many equally valid reasons for choosing one of these other providers rather than the hospice — even when someone is terminally ill. But hospice is a specific kind of care, with a specific philosophy and a rationale intrinsic to all hospice models. Based on this philosophy, a program that provides hospice services and meets hospice standards and can accurately call itself a hospice gives a different kind of care than what is offered by other health care providers promoting themselves as "just like hospice." Just because a health care agency takes care of dying patients does not make it a hospice.

However, that is not to say you can't "do it yourself" and care for a dying loved one at home without the help of hospice if you are strongly motivated to research and line up other supportive services to help in managing the care. Hospice has no copyright on principles of pain relief and palliative care, and many of these principles can still be practiced even if a formal hospice program never becomes involved. But hospice programs are structured to take much of the worry and confusion out of taking care of a terminally ill loved one.

𝕏 *Coverage for Hospice Care*

Many American hospices began as small, volunteer enterprises located in church basements or one-room offices, with rudimentary administrations and small budgets that could be supplied through community donations. Others relied on pilot-project grants from the government or from private foundations. However, as hospices grew, their permanent establishment created the need for routine, reliable sources of income to pay the salaries of professional staff. Since two-thirds of hospice patients are sixty-five years or older, naturally the place to look first was Medicare, the primary insurer for most Americans sixty-five and older.

In 1982 the U.S. Congress included a little-noticed amendment to its huge annual national budgetary statute called the Comprehensive Omnibus Budget Reconciliation Act. This amendment, authored by Democratic Congressman Leon Panetta of California, created the Medicare hospice benefit, which went into effect in November of 1983. The Medicare benefit has subsequently redefined the provision of hospice care in America and the range of services that hospices provide. It has also helped to standardize a diverse industry, as more and more hospices develop the policies and services needed to qualify for Medicare payments.

The Medicare hospice benefit was a unique political achievement for hospice advocates, and the only new federal health care entitlement to be created during the benefit-cutting first administration of President Ronald Reagan. Hospice has continued to enjoy strong bipartisan support in Congress, with sponsorship by some of the most influential members, almost yearly legislative improvements, and annual designation of November as National Hospice Month. Hospice was also an early and successful illustration of the ongoing evolution in our cost-conscious health care system away from "fee-for-service" reimbursement toward a "prospective" payment system emphasizing the health care provider's responsibility for case management.

Under the traditional fee-for-service method of health care reimbursement, every visit to the doctor's office, every visit to the home by a home care provider, perhaps even every Q-Tip or box of tissues, is billed separately, and paid at standard rates by Medicare, Medicaid, or private insurance companies. Health insurance payors may go over each submitted claim with a fine-tooth comb, looking for claims they can deny for not being "medically necessary." The provider may then turn around and bill the patient for unpaid claims, and that in a nutshell is the traditional approach to health care cost containment.

By contrast, under the Medicare hospice benefit, once the patient qualifies for the benefit, Medicare will pay the hospice provider a set rate for each day the patient is enrolled in hospice care. This is done in one of four basic per diem (daily) payment categories: routine home hospice care, general or acute inpatient care, inpatient respite care, or continuous home care for brief periods of medical crisis. Current Medicare hospice reimbursement rates, subject to regional cost-of-living adjustment, are: $86.66 per day for routine home care; $385.52 per day for acute inpatient care; $89.64 per day for inpatient respite care; and up to $505.80 for a full day of continuous home care. Out of the all-inclusive daily rate the hospice is responsible for providing — and paying the costs of — virtually every medical service the patient might require on that day. Or rather, all of those costs (plus all of the hospice's administrative overhead) get averaged out over time. The hospice nurse may spend two hours with the patient and deliver a box of supplies on Monday, while on Tuesday the patient receives only a phone call from the hospice social worker.

The traditional fee-for-service system sometimes tends to encourage health providers to give more units of service- and thus pump up their bills — although the insurance payor's claims department tries to keep an eye out for this. At the same time, the system provides few incentives to encourage effective planning or coordination between different providers and levels or settings of care, since each one submits a separate bill for its services. The Medicare approach to hospice coverage is different because the hospice pays for virtually everything the patient needs, and covers all these costs out of the flat daily rate it receives from Medicare. This approach puts a premium on effective coordination, good planning, and efficient scheduling by the hospice — in short, case management of the patient's care. It may also seem like an incentive for the hospice to provide less care under its daily rate, but in reality, since the hospice becomes financially responsible for the costs of managing expensive medical crises, it has a stronger incentive to make the patient's care run smoothly and be as trouble-free as possible. If the hospice can minimize medical flare-ups, middle-of-the-night emergencies, or rehospitalizations, it comes out ahead, financially, and so does the family, emotionally.

The Medicare benefit leaves hospices more or less free to coordinate and apportion services in ways that are most accommodating to immediate patient needs. In practice, many Medicare hospices are so successful at managing their patients' care at home, without the kinds of crises that lead to rehospitalizations, that well over 90 percent of patients' days of care are spent at home, not on an inpatient unit. Medicare also makes the hospice responsible for supervising all terminal care services which it does not provide directly. The hospice needs to have written contracts and to provide hospice training for its pharmacists, medical equipment retailers, and other ancillary service providers. Also, hospices are not permitted to discharge Medicare hospice patients just because their care has become expensive or inconvenient or has gone on too long. Only if the patient decides he or she no longer wants hospice, leaves the hospice's service area, or is no longer medically considered to be terminally ill, may a hospice discharge a Medicare patient.

The Medicare hospice benefit includes the following services: nursing care available twenty-four hours a day; medical social work; physician services; counseling; home health aides and homemakers; physical therapy, occupational therapy and speech/language pathology, when needed; medical supplies and equipment; all medications used to relieve the symptoms of terminal illness; short-term inpatient care for acute symptom management; respite for families; and continuous nursing care in the home during periods of crisis. All of the covered services should be detailed in the hospice's written plan of care developed for each patient, and approved by the patient's physician. Medicare also requires hospices to provide volunteer services, as well as bereavement support for surviving family members of deceased patients. There may be a co-payment charge to the patient of 5 percent (or $5, whichever is less) for each prescription and for each day of respite care, but this patient co-pay often is not charged to patients by hospices. The hospice benefit does not cover routine nonmedical personal supplies or grooming aids, nor does it cover the routine provision of around-the-clock maintenance care in the patient's home, since it is assumed that the family will be home watching over the patient most of the time. If the family is not able to participate in the patient's care at home, some hospices may ask the family to cover the costs of paid custodial care as a substitute for family caregivers, or else to place the patient in a nursing home.

The Medicare hospice benefit is provided to eligible patients in four benefit periods running 90, 60, and 30 days, with an indeterminate-length fourth benefit period for patients who outlive the first 210 days of benefits. At the beginning of each benefit period the patient's terminal prognosis, projected at six months or less to live, must be reconfirmed by the doctor. If a patient decides to drop out of the hospice benefit, the remaining days of the current benefit period expire, but the patient can later re-enroll, starting a new benefit period. The use of these benefit periods means, however, that there are only a limited number of times that a Medicare patient can revoke the hospice benefit and still be able to reinstate it later. With the indeterminate-length fourth benefit period, hospice coverage will continue as long as the enrolled patient still needs it and is still considered to be terminally ill, even though such a patient will have outlived the doctor's original prognosis of six months or less to live.

Because Medicare is paying the hospice a flat daily rate to cover nearly all costs of care related to the terminal illness, patients, in signing onto the hospice benefit, must waive most of their other Medicare benefits, except for doctor's visits and for certain treatments that can be shown to be unrelated to the terminal illness. Traditional Medicare benefits are reinstated immediately if the patient signs off the hospice benefit. In practice this means the hospice assumes much of the responsibility for deciding what is covered, and power to say no to covering certain services or treatments — although most Medicare hospices in fact provide virtually everything that is needed to manage the patient's care. Therefore a patient shouldn't miss any "waived" traditional Medicare benefits when enrolling in hospice, if he or she is in fact terminally ill and beyond seeking curative treatments. The ability to visit one's primary physician, and his or her ability to be paid for services by Medicare, should not be affected by enrollment on the hospice benefit.

Generally, long-term inpatient care is not provided under the hospice benefit. Nor will the hospice agree to pay for high-tech treatments that have a curative goal or focus. Patients still seeking such treatments may or may not belong in hospice care, but they definitely do not fit the Medicare hospice benefit, with its per diem method of coverage. (In some cases Medicare patients may receive services from a hospice even when they are not signed on to the Medicare hospice benefit.) Treatments such as radiation therapy, which sometimes have the goal of enhancing the patient's physical comfort, may be covered under the hospice benefit. High-tech equipment, such as continuous-drip morphine infusion pumps, may also be covered if less-intensive methods of drug administration, for example, liquid oral morphine, fail to bring adequate relief. Generally hospices exclude, either by policy or by practice, invasive medical treatments like parenteral nutrition provided through an IV line, regularly scheduled blood transfusions, or certain applications of IV antibiotics. The important issue, however, is the goal of the proposed medical treatment, and if a treatment is reasonable and necessary and it has a contribution to make to the patient's immediate physical comfort, it should be appropriately covered by the hospice under the Medicare benefit.

The patient's doctor and the hospice team will work in tandem to answer these questions about whether or not treatments are palliative and thus covered by the hospice benefit. Some patients have been put off by certain terms of the Medicare hospice benefit (as were certain hospices in the first years after the benefit's enactment): for example, the requirement for a prognosis of six months or less to live and the necessity of waiving traditional Medicare benefits when electing hospice. But in reality the hospice benefit can be a boon for those Medicare patients who are truly seeking comfort care rather than cure. The hospice becomes legally and financially responsible for providing such patients with all the care they really need, and both physicians and Medicare regulators are most interested in making sure the hospice does exactly that. A broader range of concrete services for the terminally ill are covered fully, or with only a minimal co-pay, by the Medicare hospice benefit than by traditional Medicare coverage. Patients and families may find, once the benefit is explained, that the possibility of free medical equipment and supplies, free home health aide visits, and nearly free prescriptions is more important to them than the hospice philosophy or questions it raises about medical prognosis and treatment goals.

According to the National Hospice Organization's latest census, 60 percent of the patients served by certified hospices in 1990 were covered by the Medicare hospice benefit, 4 percent were covered by Medicaid, 19 percent were covered by private health insurance plans, and most of the rest either had other Medicare coverage (for example, home health care), paid out-of-pocket, or were indigent patients (meaning they lacked either insurance or the ability to contribute personally to the cost of their care). Although Medicare, as the nation's biggest health insurance payor, often provides the lead for other insurers to follow, each private health insurance company is free to set its own policies and devise its own benefit structure. When it comes to covering hospice care, that's pretty much what has happened: each company has devised its own hospice benefit package.

A few trailblazing insurance companies and self-insured employers, starting with Connecticut General Life Insurance and General Electric in 1980, began covering hospice care even before passage of the Medicare hospice benefit. Most insurance companies have been slower to jump on the hospice bandwagon, but the trend is clearly in that direction. For instance, a Wyatt Company survey of employer health plans showed coverage of hospice rising from 15 percent in 1982 to 41 percent in 1984 to 55 percent in 1986 and still climbing. Federal Bureau of Labor statistics from 1990 show that 51 percent of health plans provided by small establishments (100 employees or less) covered hospice, as did about half of state and local government workers' health benefits, while in the 1989 survey 42 percent of medium and large firms covered hospice. However, whether or not an insurance company or health plan offers a hospice benefit for beneficiaries is only the first question to ask about insurance coverage. Since many hospice benefits are optional to the purchaser (the employer who sponsors and pays for the health insurance), the employer may need to specifically request the optional hospice benefit before it becomes available to workers. The next question is *how* hospice is covered, and whether the insurer's claims representative is willing to negotiate flexible coverage arrangements with your hospice provider.

A 1988 survey of forty-seven private insurance plans by the Joint Commission on Accreditation of Healthcare Organizations showed wide diversity in both coverage and payment levels for hospice care, with lifetime benefit ceilings ranging from $2,000 to $10,000, and even then with variations in terms of which services counted toward the lifetime ceiling. Generally, private insurers with hospice benefits utilized the traditional fee-for-service model, paying for each health professional's visit to the home, each day of hospitalization or each treatment in the hospital, and each ancillary service — rather than the all-inclusive per diem approach favored by Medicare. Private insurance hospice benefits often tended to be simply extensions or repackaging of the company's traditional coverage schedule for hospital care, home care, and other services. However, since American hospices find the per diem payment approach more appropriate to their philosophy of care, some of them are now actively pushing private insurers to adopt per diem coverage modeled on Medicare.

What if the insurance company, or your insurance plan,

doesn't cover hospice care? In many cases some or most of the *services* a hospice provides will still be covered by the insurer even if hospice care is not covered by name. Insurance companies may pay separately for regular nursing or social work visits, shifts by aides or nurses, hospitalizations, medical equipment, or other pieces of the hospice program, although they vary widely in which pieces will be covered and in requirements for "medical necessity." Because hospice patients are not going to recover, and because hospice tries to emphasize a low-tech, high-touch approach to care, some insurance claims departments will automatically call such care "custodial" and thus uncovered.

Increasingly, hospices and insurers are finding another avenue for arranging coverage, through the insurance company's individualized or large case manager. Many companies have recognized that their traditional benefit schedules don't always offer the best and least-expensive care to the individual beneficiary, especially for patients with serious illnesses and complicated needs. Instead, an individualized plan of treatment developed by the insurance company's case manager, in consultation with health care providers, can include unusual services not in the basic benefit schedule — if these alternate services are better for the patient *and* cheaper for the company. Hospices make the argument that if the insurance company case manager would give them a free hand to manage the terminally ill patient's care, at the Medicare all-inclusive rate of around $86 a day, then they could use this coverage to manage the patient's care in the best way possible in order to minimize crises and rehospitalizations. Without hospice's comprehensive approach the alternative may be for the patient's physical condition to deteriorate, resulting in a lengthy stay in the hospital at up to $1,000 a day. The logic is impeccable, though the argument has not yet been statistically proven to the satisfaction of some insurance companies. The U.S. insurance industry is gradually coming to view hospice as cost-effective generally, if not in every case or for every company.

Negotiations with insurers can be complicated. Fortunately, hospices have staff trained in working with insurance companies. Hospices will ask their patients for the name and telephone number of the insuror, and then call the company to authorize coverage for hospice care. If the insurance company offers a benefit, the hospice will utilize it. If the company has a case manager, the hospice will negotiate with that person. If the company refuses to cover hospice services in any form, it may be necessary to try alternate approaches, such as through the insurance company's complaints office, the employer's benefits manager, a union representative, or the insurance agent, to try to work out a plan for the care to which the patient is entitled. In most cases, however, if the patient has any private health insurance the odds are pretty good that it will cover hospice care one way or another.

Health maintenance organizations (HMOs) tend to include hospice care even more often than traditional insurance plans: 83 percent of respondents to a 1990 survey by the Group Health Association of America said they covered hospice. With their emphasis on case management and medical coordination, HMOs are more likely to see hospice care as a natural extension of overall managed health care and cost containment. And as the insurance industry comes to place increased emphasis on better coordination of health care services, hospice's role can only grow. The country's largest HMO, Kaiser Permanente health plan, based in Oakland, California, now offers hospice services at many of its medical centers. Ask your personal physician or HMO representative for more information.

But what if the patient has no insurance? First, hospice social workers will check to see if there are any benefits for which the patient could qualify that haven't yet been applied for. Low-income patients, for instance, may qualify for Medicaid in their state. Hospices will also ask patients and families about their financial means and ability to contribute financially to the costs of their hospice care, usually on some kind of income-based sliding scale. Because of all the over-head, coordination, and teamwork that go into hospice care, it is not cheap. The full cost of hospice care at home, whether paid per day at around $86, or per nursing visit at $70 to $100 or more, is likely to be beyond the out-of-pocket reach of most Americans for any extended period of time, and inpatient care costs even more. Hospices recognize this problem, and as a result, their sliding fee scales for self-payment are likely to request only modest contributions from most families.

In recent years it has become more common for hospices to send bills to patients for care which is not covered by insur-ance. The rationale for this policy is that if people are finan-cially able to contribute to the cost of their care, then it is reasonable to ask them to do so. Also, it is believed that if pa-tients themselves were not liable for the costs of their care, then insurance companies might feel they should not be responsible for paying, either. However, you should not let this policy deter you from contacting a hospice. If a patient can't pay, hospice managers are anxious to work out arrange-ments that will allow him or her to receive the needed care, regardless of financial circumstances. Many hospices have uncompensated-care funds to help with this.

Patients without insurance also tend to lack the ability to pay for their care, and thus hospices must care for them as in-digents, drawing upon community donations to subsidize the care. Hospices as a rule will admit patients even if they are indigent, so long as they meet other admission policies. From early in its history, the American hospice movement has believed that dying patients should not be turned away from care just because of an inability to pay for it. The National Hospice Organization's "Standards of a Hospice Program of Care" state: "To the maximum extent possible, the hospice program will admit patients regardless of their...ability to pay for services." If you are concerned about financial or coverage issues, go ahead and talk to the hospice. In most cases it will find a way to work with each individual's circumstances, to make sure all dying patients get the care they need, no matter what. A hospice that is unwilling to do this is not one to which you would want to entrust the intimate care of a dying loved one.

"With Medicare coverage, the patient often will get no bill whatever from hospice," explains James Ewens, director of Milwaukee Hospice Home Care. "Occasionally people must hire shifts of night help on their own, but even then hospice covers most of that under limited circumstances." When it comes to families with no insurance coverage, "we tell them up front, 'We will bill you, but don't worry about it.' It would be foolish not to send the bill if somebody can afford to pay it. But if they have trouble, we say, 'If you can pay a little or none, we understand. Maybe you might think of us for memorial donations.'" Ewens says. "The bottom line is that we — like most hospices — provide all of our services on the basis of patient need rather than ability to pay."

🎋 *Questions Consumers Can Ask a Hospice*

There are a number of other questions potential consumers of hospice care might want to ask a hospice program before they let this team of strangers into their homes and their lives. The hospice's licensure, certification, or accreditation can provide some assurance that it is a credible and reliable provider. But one should also ask about the hospice's admission policies and see how well they fit the individual's situation. How flexible is this hospice in applying its policies to each patient or negotiating over differences? If the hospice imposes up front a lot of conditions that don't feel comfortable, that may be a sign that it is not going to be a good fit.

How does the hospice respond to the very first call? Do telephone staff convey an attitude of caring, patience, and competence from the first contact, even if they need to ask the intake coordinator to return the patient's call? Do they speak in simple language, or do they use a lot of jargon about the requirements that patients must meet? How a hospice responds to that first call for help may be a good indicator of the kind of care to expect. If you're not certain whether your loved one qualifies for hospice — or whether you even want it — is the agency willing to make an assessment visit to help clarify these issues?

How quickly can the hospice initiate services? What are its geographical service boundaries? Can the hospice respond to unusual needs, such as putting in a telephone line for families who don't have one already but need one in order to manage the patient's care at home? Does the hospice offer specialized extras such as rehabilitation therapists, pharmacists, dieticians, family counselors, or art therapists when these could improve the patient's comfort? Are any of these extras likely to be needed in your case? Does the hospice offer to lend used medical equipment, audiovisuals, or other items that might also enhance patients' quality of life?

Ask what its policies are on inpatient care, where such care is provided, what the requirements are for an inpatient admission, and how long patients ordinarily can stay — especially if you think the patient's situation is likely to require a lengthy inpatient stay. Find out what the average length of stay is on the inpatient unit, and what happens to patients who no longer need inpatient care but can't return home. If the hospice has its own inpatient unit or residential facility, you may want to request a tour, although there is little value in touring a home care hospice's administrative offices. If the patient needs to go back to the hospital, which hospitals contract with the hospice for inpatient care? Families also need to know what kind of follow-up the hospice provides for its patients when they are in the hospital, if it doesn't operate an inpatient unit itself. Does the hospice have a residential facility, or contractual agreements with nursing homes, in order to provide a safe setting of care for patients who can't be at home? Find out which nursing homes contract with the hospice, and how much of a difference the hospice actually makes in the lives of their terminally ill residents. Does the hospice provide as much nursing, social work, and aide care for each patient in the nursing home as it does in patients' own homes?

You'll want to know whether the hospice requires a family primary caregiver as a condition of admission, and if so, how much responsibility is expected from that family caregiver. What help can the hospice offer in coordinating and supplementing the family's efforts, or filling in around job schedules, travel plans, or other responsibilities? If a patient lives alone, what alternatives can the hospice suggest?

You may also want to look into the hospice's relationship with the patient's doctor, and the doctor's past relationship with the hospice. Has your doctor referred other patients to hospice recently, and was the experience a positive one? Can they work together comfortably, or should you expect conflicts? You should ask whether the hospice medical director will visit patients when this is appropriate.

It may also be worth asking who provides nursing on-call coverage for the hospice, and what their qualifications are. How accessible are they? How does the hospice respond to after-hours emergencies? A hospice that only uses an answering machine for handling medical emergency calls after hours will probably have a hard time responding to emergencies. Although operator-staffed answering services can get very busy at times, if there is always a long wait to get emergency calls answered, or if there is a busy signal or disconnection, that, too, is a problem. Remember that when you call the hospice after hours and reach its answering service, the operator must then contact the on-call nurse at home or by pager, perhaps even getting the nurse out of bed. Such a process can take ten to twenty minutes or more, but there should always be a nurse accessible this way, and that nurse should be willing to come to the home quickly if the medical situation warrants.

How frequently do the nurse and social worker come to the patient's home for routine visits? What is the average length of nursing visits? Will it be the same nurse for every visit? What is the average caseload carried by each nurse? The fewer patients a nurse manages, the more time and energy there will be for each case. Hospice nurses who have to manage more than twelve to fourteen cases may find themselves having to cut corners, just to keep up. How often will the home health aide or personal care aide visit if the patient's physical care needs are heavy? The hospice's willingness to provide extra aide shifts to help the family through rough spots is one of the best indicators of its commitment to truly meet the patient's needs. Does the hospice guarantee to provide scheduled aide services, even if the person originally scheduled for that visit calls in sick or fails to show up?

It may also be important to know whether the hospice has policies excluding treatments such as enteral or paren- teral nutrition, blood transfusions, radiation therapy, chemo- therapy, antibiotics, dialysis, ventilators, resuscitation — or anything else that might figure prominently in your care needs. This may or may not pose a problem, since some pa- tients seek out hospices to help them *get off* dialysis, ventila- tors, or other invasive treatments. However, each hospice defines covered palliative services in its own way, and some are more or less restrictive in the kinds of treatments which are excluded from hospice coverage.

Ask about the actual out-of-pocket costs for hospice care, if any. If you have Medicare or private insurance, what additional charges might there be? Does the hospice accept Medicaid? Will the hospice accept insurance "assignment," meaning that it will settle for whatever the insurance com- pany offers as payment in full, without asking the family to make up the difference? Will the hospice handle all the billing and paperwork or negotiate on the patient's behalf with the insurer? If there is no insurance, how do they handle that? Are fees charged per visit, per day, or some other way? Do they have a sliding fee scale, or a payment plan? Will they care for patients who have no ability to pay for the care as cheerfully and as thoroughly as they do for paying clients?

"If I were a consumer and I lived in a community with more than one hospice, I would shop for a program flexible enough to see me as the individual that I am," says Lourdes Hospice's Elaine Cox. "And were they not able to do that, I would run from them, not walk, because true hospice care has to be individuals who care for individuals. It can't just be lip service. We look at that with employees when we hire them. We have ninety patients in this hospice, and I tell our staff that when we go into their homes, we're playing by ninety sets of rules."

🎗 *Barriers to Hospice Access*

Even when a person is willing to accept the hospice approach, there may still be barriers that stand in the way of obtaining needed hospice services. Some of these barriers relate to the American hospice movement's youth and growing pains and may be worked out in the future. Most hospice programs started out small and grew slowly so that they could be sure the care they did provide was of high quality, even if that meant not being able to serve everyone who wanted it. Even to start a hospice program required highly motivated individuals who were willing to put in long hours at no pay to do the necessary organizing. Hospices were not always able to hire staff or build facilities fast enough to meet the demand for their services. Some used a waiting list when they reached what they perceived to be full capacity—which is understandable, but unfortunate, since people on hospice waiting lists tend to die before they can reach the top of the list.

Hospice care is not currently available in every locality, and those areas that are not served tend to be rural, geographically isolated or some distance from an urban center that might provide a base for hospice services, or in inner-city neighborhoods. In some states, including Kansas, Kentucky, North Dakota, and South Carolina, the state association of hospices has made a concerted effort to extend geographical access to hospice care across more of the state. This is done either by persuading existing hospices to expand their service areas, or by supporting the formation of new grass-roots hospice organizing committees in unserved communities. Other hospices have grown by establishing satellite offices and teams in communities too far away to be reached by staff from the hospice's central office.

The problems faced by hospices in rural areas include long distances that must be driven by staff to reach patients' homes, sometimes on unpaved roads; difficulty finding qualified professional staff in rural areas; and the low population density that limits program efficiency. A hospice serving five patients may have many of the same overhead expenses as one serving forty patients, but it doesn't have the ability to spread these as widely, which means that the cost of caring for each patient will be higher. Rural health care in general is facing a crisis today, with many rural hospitals having to cut back or close. And if the nearest hospital is fifty miles away, that can pose additional problems for hospices trying to deal with emergencies in the patient's home. In remote areas, such as the Alaskan outback, the delivery of hospice care in the patient's home may even depend on bush pilots.

Yet a number of American hospices have found ways to thrive while serving geographically dispersed areas. Hospice of Southern Illinois in Belleville serves twenty-six largely rural Illinois counties using a toll-free 800 telephone number and fax machines to facilitate its communication and medical charting. Rice Hospice in Willmar, a town of eighteen thousand people in southern Minnesota, has four satellite offices covering territory up to 140 miles from its main office. Part-time employees and volunteers staff these satellite offices, while Rice Hospice's core management staff are on the road three days a week, car-pooling from Willmar to the satellite towns. Heart of the Hills Hospice in Kerrville, located in the wide-open spaces of west Texas, supplies company cars to its staff personal care aides so that they can reach the homes of patients in a fifty-five-mile radius from the hospice's office.

If your community does not have a hospice, someone

needs to step forward and begin the laborious process of organizing one. Help is available from the National Hospice Organization, from your state's hospice association, from existing hospices in neighboring communities, and from numerous leaders of the American hospice movement who are committed to providing advice and even in-person consultation to new hospices, often at no charge or for only the cost of travel expenses.

A problem similar to the lack of access in rural areas is the inadequacy of hospice services or access in some inner city neighborhoods — and for similar reasons: limitations in the services of the larger health care system and the absence of people willing and able to step forward and organize hospice services. As a result, American hospices today report that they tend to serve a population of patients that is disproportionally white, middle-class, and suburban.

National Hospice Organization President John J. Mahoney says that the proportion of minorities served by hospices has improved in recent years. The 1990 national hospice census shows that 14 percent of patients served by Medicare-certified hospices and 11 percent of patients served by noncertified hospices were people of color. African-Americans accounted for 8.6 percent of Medicare-certified and 7.5 percent of noncertified hospices' patients. In the previous year's census only 11 percent of hospice patients were people of color, although one in five Americans is nonwhite. Since people of color have equal or higher incidences of hospice-appropriate illnesses such as cancer and AIDS, clearly they are not receiving a proportionate share of America's hospice services.

Audrey Gordon, of the University of Illinois at Chicago School of Public Health, has examined this issue in depth, and she estimates that African-Americans who died of cancer in 1987 and 1988 were "underserved 22 percent in proportion to the cancer deaths in the hospice population when compared to the population as a whole." Similar disparities also exist among hospice employees, hospice volunteers, and hospice boards of directors.

Other minority groups may be even less likely to have access to hospice care because of language or cultural barriers. Even when hospice staff and dying patients share a common language, cultural differences in attitudes toward illness, medical care, and dying can make it difficult for some patients and families to understand or appreciate what hospice has to offer. In some traditional Japanese families, for instance, informing a loved one that he or she has a terminal illness would be unthinkable. The hospice approach might also seem at first glance like second-class medicine or "less care" to people who lack adequate health insurance or have depended on overcrowded public hospitals and clinics for their medical care. Hospice staff coming into insular minority communities and offering to help people die more comfortably may also be mistrusted as "do-gooders."

In recognition of the need for hospices to take a more proactive stance in improving access to hospice care by currently underserved minority communities, the National Hospice Organization created a Task Force on Access to Hospice Care by Minorities, chaired by Bernice Catherine Harper, of the Health Care Financing Administration. This group sponsored an open community forum in an inner-city Detroit church during NHO's November 1990 annual conference and, in June of 1991, a Washington, D.C., conference of national and local minority health advocacy groups to introduce hospice concepts and establish liaisons with these groups. The task force is also translating a generic hospice brochure into a number of different languages.

When Carolyn Fitzpatrick-Cassin became executive director of Hospice of Southeastern Michigan, she was challenged by a board member who said, "'I don't believe you have a commitment to minorities.'" This hospice's main office is in suburban Southfield, but it serves three counties in and around urban Detroit. The board member, Wilson Copeland, a prominent Detroit attorney, even threatened to resign from the hospice's board of directors, and he challenged the hospice to "do something different." "The hospice board agreed that he was right, and then challenged Wilson Copeland to help us find the best minority staff for our hospice," Fitzpatrick-Cassin says.

As a result of Copeland's challenge, the Michigan hospice set goals for improving minority access, established a task force, and studied what other hospices had done. "In June of 1990 we kicked off our Detroit hospice team, which today has a census of ninety-six patients. Our inner city team is unique," Fitzpatrick-Cassin says. "It has a different mix of staff, more social workers and home service aides, and we even have a funeral director on staff because people in the community say they want assistance with funeral planning. Another thing, we have gotten involved politically with the Detroit mayor's office, and have integrated ourselves into the social service fabric of the city. We even hired a community liaison person just to work with the city of Detroit."

For other hospices to adequately serve minority populations will require similarly intensive efforts, Fitzpatrick-Cassin says. "You have to make a commitment. It has to be of paramount importance to your staff, board, and administration." What's been the result of the effort in Detroit? Hospice of Southeastern Michigan in 1991 served a caseload that was 23 percent African-American, with roughly 1 percent each Asian-Americans and Hispanics, a 25 percent nonwhite proportion that almost exactly matched the population of its service area.

When Congress passed the Medicare hospice benefit, hospice became a public entitlement for all Medicare beneficiaries, the same as any other type of covered health care. As more insurance companies and health maintenance organizations make hospice a covered benefit, hospice providers will be challenged even more to make this benefit accessible to all who might need and want it — regardless of historical barriers to hospice access or past patterns of service that tended to favor a white, middle-class clientele. In trying to better serve minorities, hospices are also challenged to make sure their boards of directors, staffs, and volunteers reflect the cultural diversity of the communities they serve — and to develop closer working relationships with the institutions that already serve minority communities, such as the churches. American hospices are now recognizing this issue as a problem — but will they do the hard work necessary to solve it?

Speaking to hospice administrators at the 1991 NHO annual meeting, Bernice Harper said, "As much progress as we've made, I believe we've only touched the surface. . . . We have to be able to open up and see there are needs (for hospice care) beyond what we're already doing. Is hospice as good as we say? If hospice is to help people live with dignity until they die, then the minority community is wide open to you."

🕸 *Beverly*

After Beverly Thielman found out that her husband Don had incurable melanoma, she continued working at her new job, but with reduced hours. The decision to enroll in hospice meant no more visits to the cancer clinic to see Don's physician. "So we got from hospice that one-on-one, professional, physical caregiving, where he was being monitored regularly by the nurses, who kept in touch with the doctor. As far as medications, whatever, they kept track of what he needed, and didn't need, as changes occurred. That was vital, because this could all be done in our home, in a very loving environment, rather than with hospitalizations and trips to the doctor," Beverly says.

"I deeply appreciated the help with housekeeping, because it wasn't just housekeeping, it was staff who would come and visit with Don and hold his hand, and get to know him, and talk. Then they would go do the laundry," which was increased because of his illness-caused incontinence. This support from the hospice home health aide was invaluable because it freed Beverly up to spend more quality time with her husband.

How hard is it to care for a dying loved one at home? "It's hard. There's nothing easy about it, because everything is an admission that you're going to be alone. The love that you had is going to be absolutely gone. As I cared for him, and knew he was dying, every day I was letting go of a few more things." Don's physical care was also a burden. "Some of it could have been horrible, but we would turn it into something hilarious. When he became incontinent, there were times we turned it into a shower together," Beverly says.

"What I saw happen was that the HospiceCare folks encouraged me and encouraged Don to reminisce a great deal, and to talk about the life that he had lived, the life that I was yet to live, and there was always a sense of celebration in that — it was the craziest thing." During his illness, Don read a lot, enjoyed visits from the children of his first marriage, "and said a lot of farewells. Fortunately, he knew the time limitations he had in life. A lot of people don't have that. He was able to close his life here in a lot of good ways. The telephone was beside him at all times, and he called people frequently," Beverly recalls. "We also talked a lot. My office hours were shortened, and when I came back home, I would get into loungewear, and we'd both curl up on the hospital bed together and talk and talk and talk. They were very precious times, and I would encourage that for people who accept hospice into their lives, to really appreciate those moments, because they're treasures to me now. We created a lot of memories together."

CHAPTER SEVEN

Pain and Physical Realities

What is palliative care? It is attention to detail.
— Balfour Mount, M.D.,
*founder of the Royal Victoria Hospital Palliative Care
Service, Montreal, Canada*

*Is it easy? No. I've taken care of dying family members at home,
and no, it's not easy. But if it's something they want, and if the person wants to do it for them, it's going to work. It really will.*
— Michele Glass,
*patient care coordinator, Hospice of Hope,
Maysville, Kentucky*

For the patient, a terminal illness is a gradual physical deteri-
oration or decline, a kind of wasting away accompanied by a
variety of physical symptoms, manifestations, and discomforts. Dying has been described as a series of losses in every
facet of the person's existence. People with terminal illnesses
lose their jobs and countless other social roles, their independence, personal relationships, and control over countless
other aspects of their lives, even control over their bowels
and bladder. Along the way body image and self-image also

change, calling into question the person's very identity: who am I, now that I can't work, or walk, or bathe myself anymore? After all these other losses comes the final one — loss of life.

Among the nitty-gritty physical realities of a terminal illness such as cancer, the most significant is pain. Pain is a universal, and universally dreaded, experience, and unbearable pain and suffering are central to the public's conception of what it means to have a terminal illness. The pain associated with cancer is described with words such as agonizing, cruel, crushing, excruciating, grinding, ravenous, suffocating, or wrenching. In reality, one-half to two-thirds of cancer patients report pain. All but a very few of them could enjoy significant relief from their pain — if their medical professionals were dogged enough in pursuing a medical solution for it. Pain is a complex phenomenon, and treating it requires skill and persistence. But treating pain is what hospices do best.

Pain is a subjective experience, defined in the perception of the individual, but that doesn't mean it isn't very real. The pain messages that the nervous system sends to the brain are interpreted in light of personal factors such as age, sex, cultural background, and past experience with pain — as well as what the pain means to the person. Pain can provide useful and even life-saving information by telling us that something is wrong in our body and that we need to do something about it — quickly. But what if we can't do anything about it? What if it is caused by a tumor that can't be cured? The body continues to give the urgent message that something is wrong, but we can't act on that message. In time the pain is transformed from a useful message to a serious medical problem in its own right. If the pain is severe enough, it may come to fill the patient's entire waking life, with every bit of energy spent trying to escape, deflect, or otherwise cope with it.

Medical researchers draw a distinction between *acute pain* — which is sharp, localized to a physical source, and limited in duration — and the *chronic pain* that accompanies advanced cancer. Chronic pain is not limited in duration; it becomes a constant companion. With no hope for its end, it comes to dominate the future with the dread of more pain, as well as the memory of past pain. This distinction may seem like a truism — chronic pain lasts longer than acute pain — but in fact there are measurable physiological differences between the two. A severe acute pain may be accompanied by dilated eyes, sweating, or increased respiration and heartbeat, symptoms that are not present with chronic pain. On the other hand chronic pain, which creates a sense of helplessness, is often accompanied by depression or anxiety. One can perhaps summon the strength to face an acute pain of limited duration, no matter how severe, but how can one do it for a pain that has no end in sight? Medical philosopher Eric J. Cassell, M.D., has reminded us that pain and suffering are not identical experiences, although they are related. Some people in severe pain, for example, women in childbirth, don't experience their pain as suffering, which Cassell defines as a threat to the person's integrity or sense of wholeness. Others may suffer from an attack to their wholeness even when their physical pain is not so severe.

The chronic pain that accompanies cancer has three basic sources. The first is the direct result of the tumor's growth, as it invades, compresses, or obstructs various parts of the body. A second category of pain is from the side effects of medical treatments such as surgery, chemotherapy, or radiation therapy. The third type of pain is coincidental, or a byproduct of the illness. For example, a bedbound patient may develop painful bedsores from lying in one position too long. These sores are not directly caused by the cancer, but they would not have happened if the person weren't ill.

Hospice professionals have developed a number of principles of pain relief, built on the foundation of pioneering English hospice physicians such as Dame Cicely Saunders and Richard Lamerton, M.D., but refined in light of new pain research. The first principle is that only the person with pain can say whether pain is present, and how severe it is. If patients say they are in pain, then they are in pain, and they should be treated accordingly. Health professionals need to identify the source of pain, if possible, because that will influence the choice of treatment. Multiple sources or causes of pain are not unusual, but each pain deserves its own medical treatment. Physical sources of pain should be addressed first, but it should also be remembered that physical pain is intimately connected to emotional, psychological, and spiritual factors — in other words, the patient's total experience of pain. Hospices are "challenged not only to alleviate the pain of cancer, but also the 'pain of dying,'" says English hospice physician Derek Doyle, M.D., (in *Palliative Care: The Management of Far Advanced Illness*).

Careful assessment of pain is essential. Hospice patients can use a body chart to pinpoint where their pain is located and a numerical scale to rate their pain from 0 to 10. Because people are often discouraged from complaining, they may need reassurance that their pain will be taken seriously. Continual reassessment is also important, and the dosage of pain medication must be adapted and frequently modified to the individual's needs. The least intrusive method of drug administration (generally, by mouth) that is still effective is the preferred route; and the lowest dose or least powerful medication that still relieves the pain is preferred. But if a milder medication fails to control the pain, the professional's next step is to try something stronger.

It is better to prevent chronic pain, when possible, than to treat it each time it reappears. Medications for severe pain need to be given on a regular schedule (for example, every four, six, eight, or twelve hours), twenty-four hours a day, rather than just as needed. Patients and families should be educated about the goals of pain treatment and why it is essential that pain medications be given on schedule around the clock. The effect of around-the-clock administration, which keeps a constant minimum level of pain medication in the bloodstream, is that the patient can now stop worrying about the pain, relax, and even sleep. Often the medication dosage can then be cut back to a lower maintenance level, once the vicious cycle of pain and fear of pain has been broken.

The potential side effects of pain treatment should also be anticipated and aggressively treated. Constipation is such a common effect of morphine that hospice physicians may prescribe a stool softener as a preventive measure in virtually every case. Morphine-induced nausea and other common side effects are also relatively easy to treat. Generally, morphine will cause sedation for the first few days, but the patient may just be catching up on lost sleep. Usually it is possible to return the patient to a conscious, alert condition once the optimal dosage of medication has been established. The common fear that morphine will cause respiratory suppression is not a real problem for most hospice patients. In those few cases, very close to the end, when pain medications might seriously slow down the patient's breathing, hospice still recommends making relief of pain the primary medical goal. Some patients also fear that if they take morphine for moderate pain problems, they'll have nothing left to treat the severe pain they expect will come later. This fear is unwarranted. Extremely high doses of morphine that might kill another person are easily tolerated by someone with severe chronic pain. Pain is described as a narcotic antagonist and in a very crude sense the morphine is "used up" in fighting the pain.

Hospice experience also insists that the fear of narcotic addiction, dependence, or tolerance is simply not appropriate when it comes to relieving pain in dying cancer patients. This is not just because they are dying, although it makes no sense to deny pain relief to someone who is dying out of a fear that they might be addicted in the future. In fact, cancer patients receiving morphine for pain relief generally do not get addicted. They are not taking the drug for the same reason as recreational users or addicts of street narcotics such as heroin, so their experience just isn't the same. There may be some tendency toward dependence with narcotic pain medications, but if the pain were to suddenly go away or the drug were no longer needed for other reasons, the dose could be gradually and safely tapered off to nothing under a doctor's care. On the other hand, when a patient is not given adequate pain relief, or else pain medications are given only on an as-needed basis, then the person can become obsessed with the drug, always thinking about the pain and watching the clock for the next dose. What cancer patients crave is pain relief — not drugs or euphoria — and if they are given adequate pain relief, their whole outlook on life changes.

Morphine is the most common pain medication for hospice patients, when the pain is too severe to respond to milder analgesics such as aspirin, Tylenol, or ibuprofen. It is highly effective in treating even the most severe pain. However, pain relief for hospice patients does not end with morphine. Other narcotic pain medications may be used in place of morphine in certain situations. These include

meperidine (brand name Demerol), methadone, levorpha-
nol, hydromorphine (Dilaudid), oxycodone (Percodan or
Percocet), propoxyphene (Darvon, Darvocet), and codeine.
There is no evidence that heroin would be any more effective
in the relief of cancer pain than morphine, which is why hospice physicians have not participated in periodic legislative
attempts to legalize heroin for medical purposes.

Depending on the type and intensity of the pain, a number of other drugs may be used as "co-analgesics," alongside
morphine or other narcotics, to enhance their effectiveness.
The doctor or hospice nurse will know when co-analgesics
are called for; they may include corticosteroids, nonsteroidal
anti-inflammatory drugs, muscle relaxants, amphetamines,
tranquilizers, antidepressants, or other mood-altering drugs.
Other medications, antibiotics, for example, might be needed
to treat conditions such as infections that are the underlying
cause of pain or distress. In cases when high doses of narcotics or drug combinations are not achieving adequate pain
relief (or else they only relieve the pain at the cost of render-
ing the patient unconscious), then other techniques need to
be tried. Continuous-drip morphine infusion pumps are frequently used to release a constant level of morphine directly
into the bloodstream when high doses are required. Small
doses of analgesics are sometimes injected directly into the
spine to have more effect on the nervous system, and in rare
cases nerve blocks or neurosurgery can be performed to control the pain.

Even these advanced techniques are not the end of the
story in hospice pain relief, however. Doyle explains: "It cannot be stated too strongly that a purely 'pharmacological'
approach, no matter how skilled, is bound to fail in many patients." For example, some tumor-induced pain might require surgery or radiation therapy. With the physician's

permission, a little Scotch or sherry might be helpful, or else application of heat or cold, massage, physical therapy, acupuncture — even hypnosis. Patients can be taught relaxation therapy, biofeedback, meditation, or other techniques that can help reduce their anxiety and thus enhance pain relief measures.

Pain researchers also understand that a patient's feelings of fear, loneliness, frustration, anger, depression, isolation, or boredom may increase his or her experience of pain, whereas if the person's emotional outlook can be improved, so will the pain relief. Insomnia and fatigue also increase pain, so a sleeping pill offering a good night's sleep can be part of a pain relief program. Sometimes just a sympathetic listener for the patient's complaints about physical and spiritual pain and suffering can be an important adjunct in pain relief. Whatever is necessary to relieve a patient's pain should be done, and if one approach fails, hospice professionals must keep at it until a successful alternative is found.

Euthanasia advocates like Derek Humphry often claim that cancer pain is intractable — meaning that it cannot be relieved — in 10 percent of cases. However, most hospice professionals dispute this number, arguing that if all of the measures outlined above are appropriately and aggressively utilized, pain can be relieved in all but a very few cases. That does not mean every bit of pain will be eliminated, but it does mean the patient should be given a level of freedom from pain and a quality of life that are acceptable to that person.

Betty C.

"Just as soon as the surgery was over, the surgeon explained to us that this was it, there was nothing more to be done. And our family doctor, who was one of the medical directors of hospice, suggested right off: 'I think you should get hospice right away,' recalls Betty Chisholm, whose husband, Fleming, died a year earlier, two months shy of their fiftieth wedding anniversary, at home and under the care of Hospice of the Bluegrass in Lexington, Kentucky.

"I sort of knew beforehand, and he did too," Betty says. "Flem had already experienced two heart attacks, and one morning he came down to breakfast and announced that he had blood in his stools. I said, 'Oh, Fleming, it's probably tomatoes.' I was hoping and trying to make it not be blood." It was cancer, but Fleming decided not to pursue chemotherapy. "Both our family doctor and the surgeon said, 'If he were my father, I don't think I'd want the treatments.' I wasn't crazy about chemotherapy anyway, so we just went along with what they said. And I have been so grateful that we did. Fleming was never back in the hospital, and he was able to be up and going and feeling good. To me, it was just not worth living another year always sick and feeling terrible. With his having one year, and having a good year, I've never regretted it. We had a wonderful life, and we had a wonderful year that last year."

Betty had some prior knowledge of hospice, "but not the whole idea. I knew it was terminal care, and that a friend of mine had had it years before," she explains. "When they mentioned hospice, even though I was prepared for it ahead of time, my feeling was, well, this is it. It sort of finalizes things," she adds. "After we came home from the hospital, I just hated to bring it up. I didn't know how he would accept it. So finally I said, 'Fleming, your doctor thinks we should get hospice. What do you think about that?' He said go ahead and call them, so I did and two of the women came out. He was still in bed at the time. They explained hospice to him and said, 'Well, do you want to think about it, or do you want to sign up now?'" He signed up right away.

"I think Flem felt we had enjoyed such a good life; we had three wonderful children, five grandchildren, and I think he was so proud of us, all of his family. Plus there was his great faith. He just accepted the doctor's recommendations. He accepted the whole thing, and we decided we'd make however long we had the best we could," Betty says. "The very day before his kidneys started going was one of his very best days," spent with five visitors. "It really surprised me how well he took things. He never got really down and discouraged," she says.

"I didn't dream hospice would be that wonderful. I knew it would be supportive, but it's amazing how they do it — I mean everything." Isn't 'wonderful' an odd choice of words, given the circumstances? "I guess you realize you aren't going to have each other forever," Betty explains. "You want to make the very best of it you can — which we should all do anyway. No one's promised forever. And if you could just live each day the best you can, what a wonderful world we would have."

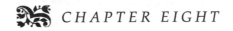

CHAPTER EIGHT

Legal Issues

In addition to the many medical and practical matters involved in caring for a dying loved one, there are some legal issues that deserve attention from both the patient and family caregivers. The extent of the patient's insurance policies and other benefits should be carefully explored. The person may qualify for certain public entitlements, such as Social Security disability benefits, social service department chore workers, Veterans benefits, Medicaid, or legal aid services. It is recommended that patients complete a will spelling out how to divide up their estate, even if it is not a large one. This can prevent problems later for families; otherwise the estate can get tied up in probate court. In some states a handwritten or "holographic" will written entirely in the patient's hand may be legally recognized, but other families may find it worth investing in the services of a lawyer knowledgeable in wills and probate. Some assets might also be legally transferred to family members before the patient's death.

If the patient is expected to die at home, there may be questions about who is legally recognized in your state to pronounce the patient dead and to sign the death certificate. Some states will allow home care nurses to pronounce death, or to consult with the physician and have the physician sign the death certificate based on a telephone conversation. Others may require a physician, coroner, or emergency medical personnel to do the actual pronouncement of death in person. It may be helpful for the attending physician to write a letter in advance stating that the patient is terminally ill and planning to die at home without life-support measures, and/or to sign an out-of-hospital do-not-resuscitate order that could be legally recognized and honored in your state. As some families have discovered to their regret after calling 911 or other emergency medical services, the first hours after the patient's home death can be much less chaotic and upsetting if they are managed without having to involve emergency personnel or police. Hospices recommend that families call them instead of 911 when the patient expires.

Another major responsibility that can be dealt with while the patient is still alive involves patient and family preferences regarding funerals, burial, or cremation. Many people have strong feelings, one way or the other, as to whether they would prefer cremation or a traditional burial, and how they want to be remembered. That is why it is important to address these questions in advance. Patients can actually choose in advance their own funeral parlor, funeral music, pallbearers, cemetery plot, and certain other preferred arrangements, or else sign up with a burial society to help simplify the arrangements. Funeral homes should be willing to give some price and other information in advance, and some may be willing to negotiate an all-inclusive rate. By shopping around, it should be possible to find a mortuary that will also agree to accommodate the family's special needs at the time of death and make suggestions about how to make transfer of the deceased person's body less traumatic. With some advance planning it might also be possible to request that funeral home personnel not use a body bag when carrying the patient out of the home for the last time. Some patients want to donate their body or body parts to medicine, which will dictate special procedures at the time of death if the body parts are to be usable. The more of these questions that can be answered in advance, the fewer decisions must be made by family members in their acute shock immediately following the death.

Advance directives are written legal documents that provide instructions for the provision of health care should the individual executing the directive become incapacitated and unable to express his or her desires about medical treatment. It is a fundamental legal principle in this country that a competent adult has the right to consent to or refuse any medical treatment. However, medical treatment decisions today have become so complicated that this right can become difficult to safeguard. There are also circumstances when, because they are physically or mentally incapacitated, patients are unable to say whether they want a treatment or not. Certain highly publicized cases such as that of Nancy Cruzan, a young Missouri woman left in a persistent vegetative state following a car accident, have made Americans more aware of the overuse of medical technology and the danger that they, too, might end up on life-support measures such as ventilators or feeding tubes, even if they were in an irreversible coma.

Advance directives such as living wills or Durable Power of Attorney for Health Care give people the opportunity to "speak" in advance for their treatment preferences when the time comes that they are no longer able to communicate. A living will lists the types of treatments a person might want or not want under certain medical circumstances — for example, no heroic measures if there is no chance for recovery. Durable Power of Attorney for Health Care allows people to express such preferences *and* to name a trusted friend or relative to speak on their behalf about treatment decisions, should they become incapacitated.

Although living wills and other advance directives have become popular in the wake of the Cruzan case, ethics experts warn about the limits to their usefulness. It is hard to anticipate in advance what medical circumstances might arise, so a living will may only provide crude directions in situations where more complex choices are called for. It is recommended that living wills be used to focus on the person's values, goals, and objectives for medical treatment, rather than just the specific types of treatment to be used or refused. Better yet is to have someone who can be legally recognized as your proxy, with whom you have discussed your values, and whom you can trust to represent your feelings no matter what eventualities may arise.

"Sometimes ventilators are morally required, but sometimes even changing the sheets is contraindicated," argues Joanne Lynn, M.D., a Washington, D.C., hospice physician. If incapacitated herself, Lynn would prefer family choice *over* the opportunity to make her own choices in advance, based on trust in her family to have her best interests at heart. Hospices also believe that the act of sitting down and talking about these painful issues with your loved ones can be more valuable for medical decision making than a piece of paper.

Since December of 1991, when the federal Patient Self-Determination Act went into effect, health care agencies such as hospices that receive federal funds are required to inform all patients of their rights to refuse or consent to treatments, and how to legally execute advance directives. Such information can help guide families in how to proceed with these documents if they wish to use them.

✣ *Anna Walton*

Anna Walton, the director of Hospice of Lake Cumberland in Somerset, Kentucky, describes spending eight hours one Friday with a hospice patient who had advanced liver cancer and was confined to her bed. The patient was middle-aged and had several children but had lost her husband several years before. One of her children, a teenager, was permanently brain-damaged and was staying with relatives in another state.

This patient was already jaundiced, and it appeared to Walton that she wouldn't live another month. "Her doctor had recommended that she try an experimental chemotherapy protocol, and from what I had read about that treatment, people in her advanced condition often got intractable nausea, vomiting, and diarrhea, and died within days of starting the treatment. Well, I went to see her one day with another nurse, and we spent the whole day there. My purpose in going that day was to let her know what might happen if she took that chemotherapy treatment, because she had been talking about how when she got better she was going to see her son again and watch another son graduate from college. And I just didn't think she was going to make it," Walton explains.

"We spent half the day talking about what she was

going to do when she got cured. She said, 'I've got some knitting in the living room, and I've got some crocheting in the basement. If you'll go get that, I'll show you what I'm working on for different people. And if you'll get that photo album out of the dining room, I'll show you the hair color of the girl I'm making this pretty coral sweater for.' She had all these projects started, in the closets and everywhere, ten different sweaters, which to me was like bargaining, because if she started one she might finish it, but if she had all these different sweaters started, she might live long enough," Walton explains.

"So after she went through all of that, I said, 'So you really think you're going to be cured?' She said, 'No, I know I'm dying.' But it was only after speaking for four or five hours with her that I had the rapport to ask her that. She said, 'I know I'm not going to get better.' I said, 'What do you think is going to happen?' She said, 'I know that shortly I'm not going to be alive. I've got to take this treatment in the hopes that I'll at least get to see my son again.' I said, 'I'm going to tell you what could happen if you take the treatment.' And then I asked her, 'If you knew without a doubt that you had only thirty days left to live, what would you do? What one thing would you like to do?' And she said, 'I'd like to see my son.' I said, 'Would you like me to call my friend who's a travel agent and arrange that, for you to go to him, and have hospice care where he's staying?'"

The woman went to her son, enrolled in a hospice there, and died there without taking the chemotherapy. Walton said, "I thought to myself, 'I wonder what that doctor is going to do when I tell him.' So I just went to his office and explained to him what I did and why. He was so thankful. He sees eighty to a hundred patients a day. He said, 'How could we possibly do what it took you eight hours to do?'"

CHAPTER NINE

The Place for Hope in Hospice

Hope and acceptance of death are basic concepts because they insist that mortality is a dimension of living, not merely a negation or an end-point that cancels out everything. Hope is, indeed, the basic assumption in living and dying, and it sickens in an atmosphere of persistent, ill-founded deception and denial.
— Avery Weisman,
On Dying and Denying: A Psychiatric Study of Terminality

Although hospice is care for the terminally ill, hospice professionals insist that entering hospice does not require giving up hope. They often say that the nature or the focus of hope changes when the illness is known to be incurable, and when the patient enters hospice care. Perhaps it is no longer realistic to hope for a cure. But one might still hope to live long enough to attend a fiftieth wedding anniversary, a daughter's wedding, or a son's graduation, or to be present for a grandchild's birth. One can hope to heal family rifts, to say goodbyes to loved ones coming from far away, to find peace and acceptance before the end, to get out of the house one last time, or to achieve some understanding about the meaning and purpose of one's life and death. At a more basic level of existence one might simply hope for freedom from pain, a good day today, a good night's sleep, a comfort-promoting bowel movement. But is that enough?

Hope is not something that a physician gives to you or takes away — although obviously what the doctor says can go a long way toward supporting or shaking your hope. The British psychiatrist and author Avery Weisman says hope comes from our self-image and our belief in being able to exert some control over the world around us — even though we can never have total control, so there's no such thing as absolute hope. Authentic hope, says Weisman, is not built on a desire for the impossible.

Hospices do not try to deprive dying patients of hope; in fact they see hope as essential to coping and dealing with a difficult situation. "There is a spiritual need for hope," says Hospice of Louisville chaplain J. Mark Springer. While hospice caregivers may have some suggestions about refocusing the objects of their patients' hopes, they do not try to relieve patients of the big hope — that somehow, against all odds, they might still beat the disease or benefit from a miracle cure. In fact, the hope for a cure is common among terminally ill hospice patients almost until they die. But it is also important to recognize that some hopes can be helpful and serve you well, while others can be counterproductive in trying to cope with a personal crisis such as a life-threatening illness. A willingness to talk about and explore your hopes may lead to a broader perspective about what they mean, what they can do in your life, and where they may lead.

Some people fear that accepting hospice care in their lives means giving up or throwing in the towel in their fight against the disease. They feel they must fight for life at all costs, or strive for a miracle cure. While it is true that hospice is intended for people who doctors believe will not recover, such predictions don't always come true. Some patients may live longer than their doctors expected, and a few may even get better. Medical care rarely comes with ironclad guarantees; doctors deal with probabilities. The physician may give a prediction for the patient's chances of getting better or for how much longer he or she can expect to live. But this is only a prediction, and time alone will prove its accuracy. In the meantime, with hospice's help, patients can still get their affairs in order and make any necessary plans for the worst, without necessarily relinquishing their hope that a miracle may happen.

"A primary obstacle to becoming a hospice patient has been the belief that to become a hospice patient means leaving all hope at the door," says Stephen Connor, a hospice veteran and psychologist who has studied denial in the terminally ill. "Definitely, there should be room for hope in hospice. A lot of people need to maintain a certain amount of what we call hope as they go through this experience, in order to remain somewhat sane in an insane situation," he explains. "It's not one of our admission criteria in hospice that you give up hope, although it is one of our admission criteria that you have knowledge of what is believed to be your diagnosis and prognosis. What you do with that information is your business. I tell families: 'None of us knows for sure what will happen.'" While some dying patients may fix their hopes on such reformulated goals as relief of pain, quality of life, or reconciliation with their families, most mean more than that by their hopes, and many will continue hoping for a cure almost to the end, Connor says. If they are older when they become ill, but in any case as they get closer to dying, the evidence of their medical situation gets harder to deny and the energy that they put into hoping for a cure may start to wane.

"You probably wouldn't be normal if you didn't wish [for a cure] somewhere inside," says Dana Ryan, admissions coordinator for Hospice of Central Kentucky in Elizabethtown. Adds Ryan's colleague, Donna Jones, a nurse: "I've had patients that took their last breath loving life and wanting to live." Jones describes one of her current hospice patients, a young man who one day looked her in the eye and said, "I'm not going to die." She explains, "If he's got a shred of hope, I'm sure not going to take it away. And I don't think I'm allowing him to have false hopes. We have talked about his disease process. I've answered a zillion questions for him. I think we've got enough information between us that we know where we are with this disease. I don't think he would ever say to me: 'Don't come in, I don't want to see you again because you represent death and I'm not dying.' He's not in that much denial. But on the days that he's feeling good, he goes for the gusto."

And hope — even hope for a miracle cure — needn't stand in the way of the things that can be done to better manage your situation today. On the other hand, the kind of hope that achieves a positive attitude only by shutting out all negative thoughts may not prove very useful in dealing with life's realities. William Buchholz, M.D., an oncologist in Los Altos, California, defines false hope as the creation of a perceived reality that no one from outside of the family can share, and which is so rigid it doesn't leave room for any outside assistance that might make the situation easier to manage. True hope can incorporate both positive and negative outcomes, while false hope "denies; it avoids at all costs," Buchholz explains. "If they are still coping and functioning, then their hope is well used. If the hope is separating them from other caregivers, then a problem exists."

"We've had families who believed the patient would be healed," says Julie Henahan, former director of the Elizabethtown hospice. "Our chaplains have learned to address that by saying healing may take several forms. It may not be a healing of the physical body. It may be a healing of the spirit, and we may not always be able to recognize what that healing is." Henahan's hospice recently cared for a patient whose husband believed in love, faith healing, and herbal therapy as tools to help her overcome her disease. "We didn't walk in and stop that," says Ryan. "That's one of the things he asked us about up front, and I said, 'This is what we do. What you do is what you do.'" The husband believed that if he could just find the right combination of herbs, his wife would be cured, although in the end he was not able to find it. "But I don't think it means we failed as a hospice," adds Ryan. "Nor did it make her inappropriate for hospice. She was still terminal, and we knew and the doctor knew. The husband seemed to understand that she was going to die, but he thought he could stop that."

Colleen Hoerneman, director of the Marshfield hospice, says the hospice philosophy does not discount various healing approaches. "That's the strength of hospice. I think hospice tries to look at however each individual is approaching things and whatever they may bring with them — different means of coping, different means of addressing the situation.... Whatever they bring along, that's okay," she adds. "In our hospice we've seen situations where we had maybe a Native American family for whom it was extremely important, from a ritual standpoint, to be able to do the laying on of hands or some of the other rituals that are part of that culture." Such an approach "should not only be allowed but fostered, because it is extremely meaningful, not only from the standpoint of whatever healing effect it ultimately may have, but because it also helps the family through their own grieving process," she says. "Hospice doesn't say we have the only answer. There are lots of answers, there are lots of people, and everybody is going to come to terms with their own answer a little differently. And that's okay."

CHAPTER TEN

Issues in the Future of Hospice

The community needs the dying to make it think of eternal issues.
We are indebted to those who can make us learn such things as to be
gentle and approach others with true affection and respect.
— Dame Cicely Saunders, M.D.,
founder of the modern hospice movement

If an aging and mobile society helped to shape the demand for hospice care in the 1970s and 1980s, an increasingly aged and mobile society in the 1990s will demand some modifications to the basic hospice approach. It is becoming harder for hospices to expect all or even most of their patients to have a willing, available, and reliable family caregiver in the home to do much of the patient's routine care, so hospices need to rethink their traditional requirement for a primary caregiver as a condition for hospice admission. There may not be any caregiver for elderly widows and widowers whose spouses have already died — perhaps under the care of hospice. Some very elderly patients may have a spouse, but that person, too, may be elderly, frail, or ill and thus unable to physically contribute to their care. For many broken families, single-parent households, or divorced adults living alone, there may not be anyone around to serve as the dying patient's primary caregiver. In big cities large numbers of socially isolated individuals live alone in single-room-occupancy residential hotels. The growing problem of the homeless raises questions about how to care for them, should they become terminally ill. In many families the primary caregiver can't afford to stay home from work to care for a dying loved one, or must continue working in order to preserve health insurance benefits. Caring for the growing numbers of people with AIDS will also challenge hospice's traditional notions of home and family support.

A hospice proposing today to care only for patients who can be safely managed in their own homes, with the active in-home participation of a family caregiver, will find such a policy increasingly untenable. Eventually it may even be seen as a kind of discrimination for hospices to continue serving their traditional patient profile of predominantly middle-class white patients with stable, supportive families, while turning away more needy and difficult "have-not" patients who live alone or don't have homes.

While some hospices may be reluctant to tinker with an approach that has worked well up to now for the patients they already serve, many today recognize the need for new approaches to fill unmet needs, or else have already started implementing or experimenting with various alternatives such as residential or nursing home programs. Hospices may also find organized ways to supplement or substitute for family caregivers in the patient's home with paid personal care workers, volunteers, or mobilized teams of people from the neighborhood, church, synagogue, or other community group to fill shifts at the patient's bedside.

🦋 *High Tech and Hospice*

Another important reality in the evolution of American health care demanding a response from hospices is the ongoing revolution in high-technology medicine. When hospice care first appeared in this country, it was presented as an alternative to the complex, invasive medical techniques practiced in the hospital — especially on intensive care units. Hospices were therefore reluctant to get involved with any kind of high-technology medicine, believing it to be inimical to the hospice goal of providing comfort care for dying patients.

But in the years since the first American hospice opened, there has been a revolution in medical technology, devices, and techniques. High tech has become portable, affordable, and smaller. Medical treatments formerly available only in the intensive care unit now can follow the patient home. The home-infusion-therapy industry, represented by companies such as Caremark, New England Critical Care, and T² Medical, has become a $3 billion-a-year business. Home-infusion companies provide prepared medical products in sterile plastic bags, equipment, plus necessary supervision and instruction for patients at home to receive antibiotics, blood transfusions, chemotherapy, or even nutrition intravenously. Total parenteral nutrition is a combination of protein, fatty supplements, and other nutrients that go directly into the bloodstream when the patient is unable to absorb food through the intestines. Timed-release intravenous infusion pumps make it possible to maintain a constant blood level of medications such as morphine, thus more easily controlling severe pain. Some patients now go home from the hospital with a permanent intravenous shunt, such as a Hickman catheter placed directly into a vein in their chest, enabling their physician to later prescribe other intravenous treatments when needed. Treatments for AIDS emphasize the high-tech approach even more heavily, while the technology continues to get smaller, easier to handle, and ever more portable.

The Medicare hospice benefit requires hospices to develop and implement a plan of care for the patient that provides whatever is necessary to maximize the patient's comfort; but it doesn't require covering medical treatments that contribute little to this goal. If the patient is on the Medicare hospice benefit, the hospice is required to pay for all services that are "reasonable and necessary to manage the terminal illness." What constitutes reasonable and necessary is subject to dialogue. Doctors are now trained in the use of high-tech equipment, and hospices report that some doctors will order, for example, high-tech morphine infusion pumps for nearly every cancer patient who reports pain, even when pain relief could be adequately achieved more simply with liquid oral morphine or timed-release morphine tablets. In theory it should be possible to evaluate any potential treatment for a hospice patient in terms of its goals and intentions, but in practice these can be very difficult questions to answer. When new equipment is available, there is always a temptation to use it just because it exists.

"Up to this point, hospice has been packaged as low-tech care," says Michael Levy, M.D., medical director of the Palliative Care Service at Fox Chase Cancer Center in Philadelphia, Pennsylvania. "Now we're pushing those boundaries. The state-of-the-art of hospice and home care has advanced to where we can now do things we couldn't do before. We have new capabilities, and a real pressure to take patients using these new capabilities." The problem becomes more pronounced with hydration (supplying water intravenously) and total parenteral nutrition, because of the symbolic meaning of food and fluids. Feeding the patient represents loving care to the family, while not eating signifies an imminent death. So when patients are no longer willing or able to eat, family members may demand that they be fed some other way. However, these treatments can have a number of negative consequences, adding to, rather than alleviating symptom problems, for a patient who has stopped eating in the final stages of illness. Such symptoms might include increased pain, serious edemas or swelling in the extremities, vomiting, and congestion or fluid build-up in the lungs. Whether or not to artificially feed a terminally ill patient is a question that needs to be decided by dialogue between patient, family, physician, and hospice team, on an individualized basis. However, hospices will point to a growing body of research suggesting that the provision of artificial food and fluids for someone with end-stage cancer does nothing to either significantly extend life or enhance the patient's quality of life.

ॐ *Hospice Care for People with AIDS*

AIDS (acquired immune deficiency syndrome), unknown when most American hospices were established, has become the most frightening public health crisis of our time. As this book goes to press, 242,146 cases of AIDS have been reported in the United States, and 160,372 of those people have died. But researchers estimate that an additional one million Americans may now be infected with the human immune-deficiency virus (HIV) that causes AIDS, even though many of them may not know it yet. Since there is roughly a ten-year incubation period before HIV infection develops into full-blown AIDS, and since there is no way to medically cure

AIDS at this time, most of those now infected will swell the ranks of the terminally ill in the 1990s, with horrendous medical, social, and personal consequences for this country.

If ever there were a disease that called out for the level-headed compassion and multifaceted caregiving skills of hospice, surely it is AIDS. AIDS would seem to be tailor-made for the hospice program, given its tremendous symptom-management challenges, social and emotional complications, and the fact that there is no cure. But although many hospices have provided compassionate and courageous care for people with AIDS, and a few have even taken the lead in showing their communities how to care for these people, nationwide hospices have not played as large a role in AIDS care as was once expected of them. The relationship between hospices and the service network that has developed for people with AIDS has been strained, and the reasons for this may be instructive in considering the future of hospice care in America.

Prior to the AIDS epidemic, the typical or average hospice patient was over sixty-five, lived with his or her spouse, and had cancer. Following one or more rounds of curative treatment, which proved ineffective, this patient decided to stop aggressive cancer therapy and return home with the support of hospice. Given a relatively predictable disease trajectory, the patient was considered by a physician to have six months or less to live, and in fact lived only an average of two months under hospice's care. No one would eagerly embrace such a fate, but this typical hospice patient might at least look back on a long and full life. The typical AIDS patient, on the other hand, is in his thirties or forties. Although AIDS has now spread into a larger community that includes heterosexuals, women, and children, many AIDS patients are still socially marginalized, and many are gay or bisexual men or intravenous drug abusers who all too often lack a stable and supportive family structure.

Since people with AIDS are younger, with half or more of their expected life span still unfulfilled, it is hard for them to emotionally acknowledge that their illness could be terminal, to give up on aggressive therapies, or to accept hospice care into their lives. Though AIDS treatments are not truly curative, some, like AZT, can prolong life and offer longer periods of living actively and symptom-free, while others may prevent or cure the devastating and lethal opportunistic infections that accompany advanced AIDS. The armamentarium of AIDS treatments is changing constantly, with new discoveries and a wide range of experimental drug protocols now being tested. Such treatments often have severe toxic side effects. The cumulative result of these developments is that AIDS has become more of a chronic, long-term illness than it was in its early years. Even though no cure for AIDS has yet been found, and AIDS still appears always to lead to a terminal decline, today people can live years relatively symptom-free following HIV infection, and even after they come down with AIDS. At the same time, the path of AIDS is usually unpredictable — a medical roller coaster in which a patient seemingly at death's door one week is back on his feet again the next.

Because people with AIDS are also less likely to live in safe, adequate home situations where they can receive hospice care, they often need residential or congregate living situations. If hospices don't offer such services, it will be harder for them to play a major role in AIDS care. Some hospices have developed urgently needed residential programs, or else have worked closely with other agencies that operate AIDS shelters. Visiting Nurses and Hospice of San Francisco, America's preeminent provider of AIDS hospice care, has drawn on local, state, and national funding to offer extra personal care aides and other services in the homes of its AIDS patients. When care in the home is no longer feasible, the hospice will continue following its patients in one of San Francisco's many AIDS shelters or else in its own residence program, Coming Home Hospice.

Some AIDS support agencies and advocacy groups across the country have been suspicious of hospices. They view it as a preventable tragedy that people so young are dying of this disease, and they demand a cure from government-funded research. They consider it essential for people with AIDS to fight for life with all their strength, as a political as well as a personal act, in order to still "be here for the cure." Therefore, they view entering hospice as an act of surrender. Gay leaders have also questioned the motivations and commitment of hospices and wonder whether they can respond sensitively and appropriately to the special needs of AIDS patients, who have already experienced many rejections by the system. Unfortunately, the reluctance of some hospices to boldly embrace the challenge of AIDS care, to demonstrate their goodwill, and to establish working relationships with AIDS service groups may help to fuel this mistrust. For hospices, uncertainties about the greater care needs of AIDS patients and about the increased costs of such care may lie behind their reluctance.

Hospices in San Francisco, Los Angeles, Santa Cruz, Boston, New York, Miami, West Palm Beach, and countless other cities have accepted the AIDS challenge and found ways to meet this growing need, often playing a leading role in the development of AIDS services in their communities. Some hospices have modified their admission criteria by dropping the requirement for a terminal diagnosis with six months or less to live — or else have soft-pedaled their admissions policies — in order to better serve people with AIDS. Others have developed specialized programs for people with AIDS, combining traditional hospice philosophy with new approaches and services. For example, Hospice West in Waltham, Massachusetts operates Hospice at Mission Hill in Boston, a unique eighteen-bed inpatient hospice facility for people with AIDS. VITAS Innovative Hospice Care in Miami offers care to people with AIDS through its Project Outreach, using different staffing and services than its traditional hospice teams: more inpatient care, more psychosocial support, more medications, and more high-tech services.

Early in the epidemic, Visiting Nurses and Hospice of San Francisco promoted its service as an AIDS home care *and* hospice program, blurring the distinction between these two categories of care. This was an acknowledgment of the barriers that traditional hospice policies posed for people with AIDS. Eventually its AIDS home care and its traditional hospice care for people with diseases such as cancer were combined because the similarities between these services outnumbered the differences. More recently, however, the agency has reestablished a separate "intermittent home care" service for AIDS patients who aren't yet ready for hospice.

"Our feeling, absolutely, is that AIDS patients are appropriate for hospice, but not necessarily from the moment of diagnosis, as I would have believed five years ago," says Jeannee Parker Martin, director of Visiting Nurses and Hospice of San Francisco and founder eight years ago of its AIDS hospice program. "Many patients with AIDS aggressively seek and have a goal of curative treatment, even though they have just a few months to live," she explains. "Some patients who in everybody's view but their own are appropriate for hospice, who are deteriorating and dying, still want our intermittent home care," rather than hospice.

"The question for health care consumers is at what point do they change their goals of treatment? Even if they still have a thread of hope, even if they're receiving the same drug therapies [as intermittent home care patients], even if they're still on experimental protocols, if their goal is palliation and if they understand their illness is terminal, then hospice care is the right answer," Martin says.

However, hospices report that people with AIDS are reluctant to see themselves as terminally ill, even when they are, to cease aggressive treatments even when those treatments are no longer helpful, or to accept an organization established to care for the dying. "People don't have to say 'I'm dying,' but you have to accept the hospice approach," Martin says. Does this sound familiar? These are the same issues and hurdles that can hang up cancer patients who might become potential hospice clients.

In other words, the reluctance of some people with AIDS — just like people with cancer — may have more to do with perceptions of hospice care and the symbolic meaning of hospice, than with what hospice is really about. Claire Tehan, director of Hospital Home Health Care Hospice in Torrance, California, and another pioneer in the development of hospice care for people with AIDS, says, "It has been difficult to communicate the positive aspect central to the hospice philosophy that supports their fighting spirit — the concept of the empowerment of the individual." Adds Martin, "Hospice is not only about dying. It's about living, support, guidance, and opportunities."

"We do change people's outlooks over what hospice is all about," and sometimes AIDS patients will transfer from VNHSF's intermittent home care program to hospice, Martin adds. More often, however, those AIDS patients who prefer intermittent home care stick with home care, even though they don't necessarily live any longer than the patients who are receiving the expanded support services of hospice care. Or else, says Mark Donnell, hospice team leader with VNHSF, "suddenly the patient hits the wall. Boom, they want hospice." They may then die very soon after, before hospice care can have much of an impact in their lives. "We see it week after week in the care conference: the patient is considering hospice, the family is discussing hospice. Then they hit the wall, and it turns into crisis hospice."

Visiting Nurses and Hospice of San Francisco has clearly demonstrated that hospice *can* be appropriate for people with AIDS. Eighty percent of its AIDS hospice patients are able to die at home. Its staff have learned to apply hospice symptom-management approaches to people with AIDS, even though the symptoms of AIDS can be much more challenging. The hospice has also taken its place as one of the cornerstones of the celebrated "San Francisco Model" of AIDS services, and has developed a special relationship with the local gay community, drawing on that community for staff, for volunteers, and for donations of various kinds.

However, while programs such as VNHSF have shown that hospice care is appropriate for AIDS patients who want it, there are still some key differences. The complexities and ambiguities of drug therapies can be much more difficult to sort out than for traditional hospice patients. Some AIDS drugs serve an essentially palliative purpose, for example DHPG (gancyclovir), which staves off the blindness caused by the infection of cytomegalovirus. Others, like AZT, are largely aimed at extending the patient's life span, and AZT costs $3,000 a year. Not every AIDS hospice patient ends up on a per diem Medicare or Medicaid hospice benefit, Martin says. But for those who do, the costs to the hospice are enormous. Tehan surveyed hospices serving AIDS patients and found that those covering AZT and two other common AIDS drugs, amphotericin and pentamidine, spent an average of $27 to $55 per patient *per day* on drugs alone — or one-third to one-half of their total daily reimbursement for each patient. Other estimates suggest that AIDS hospice care can cost up to twice as much as traditional hospice, but without a corresponding increase in reimbursement. This can be a real problem for the agency unless there is some additional funding source, such as a foundation grant, available. Hospices caring for AIDS patients must also deal with managing intravenous drug therapies, since that is the only way to administer many AIDS treatments. Martin says her agency does not cover experimental new AIDS drugs for AIDS hospice patients, but the rationale for this policy is the same as for not covering nontraditional or unproven services such as acupuncture.

Symptom management can be a greater challenge with AIDS patients, especially with frequent medical problems such as neuropathy or pain in the extremities, severe and persistent diarrhea, and AIDS-related dementia or confusion. Patients with AIDS are often socially isolated, and if there are friends and family members in their lives, these social relationships can get complicated. Imagine a situation in which the AIDS patient's family finds out he is gay and has a life-threatening illness, both in the same breath. Conflicts often arise between the patient's partner and the family of origin, who have been thrown together in trying to manage the patient's care. "Many of our patients today are sole survivors," Donnell relates. "They spent all of their time taking care of the people in their support network" who were dying of AIDS, and now there are no friends left to care for them. The grief of some people who have lost dozens, or even hundreds, of friends to AIDS is hard to imagine, but perhaps can be compared to that of soldiers on the front lines in wartime. This

grief of AIDS survivors can be more difficult to deal with because of the young age of the person who died, the social
stigma that makes the grief unmentionable, and the fact that
partners of AIDS patients often are themselves at risk for the
same dreadful disease.

All of these differences primarily relate to AIDS populations like the one on the West Coast, which is composed
mostly of gay men. However, the growing proportion of
AIDS patients who are intravenous drug abusers will make
all of these problems even more difficult to manage. Drug
abusers are less likely to have a home where they can receive
hospice care, which is why most hospices have only limited
experience caring for them. Compliance problems with medical care and active drug abuse will raise new dilemmas for
hospice inpatient programs. It remains to be seen whether
American hospices will find ways to care for IV drug abusers
with AIDS as many already have for gay men with AIDS.

"It's gotten harder rather than easier as we have gotten
into this epidemic," Donnell says. "Caseloads are up, support
systems are down. Originally people with AIDS had PCP
(*Pneumocystis carinii* pneumonia) and Kaposi's sarcoma. Now
they are diagnosed with five, six, and seven infections, all
currently being treated," he explains. "There are no care models; we're still making this up. We're only ten years into this
brand-new illness."

✨ Children and Hospice

Roughly 100,000 American children die every year, many
of them following an extended illness, but only 1 percent
of the 200,000 patients served by American hospices in
1990 were under the age of eighteen. In some ways the
hospice approach described in this book might be seen as

inappropriate to the parents of a young child with a life-threatening illness, since they leave no stone unturned in their efforts to find a cure for their child. They may also reject any acknowledgment that the illness could be terminal. Acceptance will prove difficult, if not impossible, when the terminally ill patient is a young child. And yet the need for emotional and spiritual support, for education and guidance on symptom management, and for assistance and resources to manage the child's care at home may be even greater than for the caregivers of older patients.

How does the hospice approach fit when the potential patient is a child? Very well, says Ann Armstrong Dailey, of Children's Hospice International, an Alexandria, Virginia–based organization established in 1983 to provide an informational clearinghouse on children's hospice care and national advocacy for making this care more widely available. "I feel really frustrated that some kids ... who are terminally ill might fall through the cracks of hospice policies, because right now hospice is the organization best equipped to deal with their needs. The difference hospice can make in these kids' lives is tremendous," Dailey insists. And yet, she points out, children with life-threatening illnesses and their parents are different from other hospice families in important ways. As for people with AIDS, modifications in hospice policies may be required if this valuable service is to be fully utilized by those who need it.

Medically it is more difficult to define a terminal phase with six months or less to live for children with life-threatening illnesses. While most adult hospice patients have cancer, with a relatively definable terminal phase, children in hospice may have a much wider variety of rare illnesses, and their terminal phase might last for years. Even when the medical picture is clear, families and doctors are understandably reluctant to recognize that a child is terminally ill or to acknowledge the crushing implications of such a prognosis. For the hospice to require such an acknowledgment may keep the parents of dying children from ever utilizing the support of hospice.

Dailey's organization, Children's Hospice International, has also identified some other key differences in hospice for children. Unlike older hospice patients, a child is not legally competent to consent to hospice care and thus depends on the parents to make all treatment decisions. The child's age and developmental process shape and limit his or her ability to understand what's happening and to verbalize needs, feelings, and desires. Parents may be overprotective in trying to shield children from the reality of what's going on. Health professionals at children's hospitals also tend to feel very protective toward "their" children, and therefore are reluctant to refer to hospices. Physicians may be unwilling to prescribe narcotic pain medications for children, and the child's different body weight and metabolism require dosage modifications for many medical treatments. If there are siblings, the family's turmoil and the parents' concentration on the sick child may cause some serious, long-lasting problems for the other children. For everyone involved in the dying child's care, the sense of failure is palpable. Insurance or public coverage for needed services, especially for home care, is often limited, which can affect the family's care choices.

Hospices, too, find caring for dying children to be more difficult, requiring more medical interventions and more psychosocial care. These cases are also stressful and painful for hospice staff, some of whom have young children of their own, and thus are able to emotionally identify with the parents' pain. At one time some hospices were reluctant to serve dying children, on the grounds that they lacked the necessary knowledge and abilities, but this picture is changing.

The most recent national survey by Children's Hospice International showed that 447 programs, or 79 percent of responding hospices, were willing to admit child patients, while 14 agencies described themselves as exclusively children's hospices. The National Hospice Organization's 1990 census shows that 95 percent of American hospices have policies that allow enrolling children as hospice patients, while 67 percent have actually served dying children.

Some hospices have developed special admission criteria for younger patients, discarding the requirement for a terminal prognosis of six months or less to live in favor of just recognizing that the child's illness is life-threatening. Others have tried to be flexible and sensitive in how their existing admission policies apply to young patients. Hospices often provide special training to staff who work with children, and develop a close working relationship with a children's hospital or medical research center, for easy access to information on rare illnesses and on symptom management.

Children's Hospice International recommends that children's hospice programs not rule out the parents' hopes for cure or desire to pursue aggressive therapies, sometimes until the very end. But instead of focusing only on cure, hospice care for children should emphasize pain and symptom management and help families deal with their fears and questions. The goal of hospice for children is "the enhancement of quality of life each day" for the patient and his or her family, however they define quality of life and whatever the eventual outcome, Dailey says. Hospice aims to facilitate communication and help the family cope better day to day. Even more than with adult patients, hospice supports and educates the parents so that they can do the caregiving. Parents will need to feel they did everything possible for their child and provided the very best care available.

What Does Choosing Hospice Really Mean?

Hospice doesn't help people die; hospice helps dying people.
— David A. Simpson,
director, Hospice of the Western Reserve, Cleveland, Ohio

"Hospice by nature is the type of program you hope you never need," says William Carter, admissions coordinator for Lourdes Hospice. "Hospice admission criteria can be a hurdle for people, a difficult thing — absolutely. That's the nature of the business. As far as getting over that hurdle, some don't get over it," Carter explains. "Most generally, it's just a resignation to the fact that this is inevitable and unavoidable. People around here are real matter-of-fact-type people. They accept the hospice referral simply as what it is: something to help you through what you're going through. Basically they're receptive to the whole idea, and by the time you explain the services to them, you get comments like: 'This is wonderful,' or 'I never realized,'" he explains.

Is there a minimum level of acceptance or understanding that patients and families must have in order to make hospice care appropriate? Marsha Sherman, oncology social worker at Saint Joseph Hospital in Lexington, Kentucky, and a frequent referrer to hospice, says there is and should be.

"The hospice philosophy is built on helping people end their lives in a dignified and respectful manner, and if that's the premise, then yes, people have to know that's why they're in the program," Sherman says. "They're in the program to get assistance living out the end of their lives. I think hospice is trying to prepare people, and just not wanting to hear about it isn't going to make it go away. Hospice has the opportunity to turn people's attitudes around and help them be accepting of what's coming, but you can't do that if you can't say it."

Basically, hospice requires an awareness of the terminal situation by the patient — without dictating what the patient's attitude toward that awareness should be. That threshhold is achieved when a patient is informed enough and open enough to recognize himself or herself as someone who can benefit from hospice's program of care for the dying. Such recognition should still allow room for an unwillingness to talk about or dwell on the fact, hope for a miraculous cure, or an intention to fight the disease with a positive attitude.

Although the word acceptance is closely linked with hospice, hospice programs don't and can't expect patients to be accepting of their dying. If hospices were to require such openness as a condition of admission, then few dying patients would qualify. It is hoped, as patients and families learn to trust the hospice team and benefit from hospice's support, that they may gradually work their way toward some kind of acceptance of or reconciliation to what is happening to them. In reality, not all hospice patients ever truly accept their dying. Some may fight or deny their fate all the way to the end, because that is how they've always lived their lives. However, it is essential that the patient and family understand what hospice is, what it offers, and what it does not provide.

Often the hospice decision is made on a purely practical basis, in terms of the patient and family's immediate needs, rather than any appreciation for the hospice philosophy. Families need advice, emotional support, assistance with caregiving chores, symptom-management expertise, and guidance in negotiating through a complicated health care system. Hospice usually is the agency best equipped to help. It's hard to imagine anyone ever warmly welcoming hospice into their lives, or elated to finally qualify for hospice services. Often the key consideration for families, says Maureen Krolikowski, a nurse with Milwaukee Hospice Home Care, is: "'How much help are you going to give us? Are you going to give us twenty-four-hour help when we need it?'"

"For some people, the fact that the Medicare hospice benefit pays for the hospital bed may be the only thing they want from us at first," although they usually end up wanting the other services, too, says Michele Glass, patient care coordinator for Hospice of Hope in Maysville. "With the wife of one patient, her first question to me was: 'I can't get my husband out of bed anymore. Would you loan me a wheelchair?' I said sure we could, and then I asked her about this and that, and told her we could help with other things and that Medicare would pay for it all. She said, 'Will you come now?'"

Resources for Families with Life-threatening Illnesses

The following is a sampling of key national resource organizations that can provide additional information to assist potential clients of hospice care, namely, people with life-threatening illnesses and their families and friends. Many of these resources could prove useful even if the patient doesn't want, or doesn't qualify for, the services offered by a hospice program. Most are available to help people from across the country with answers to general questions, printed information, and referrals to local service providers. The 800 numbers are toll-free to callers.

Consumer Information

National Consumers League
815 15th Street NW
Suite 928-N
Washington, DC 20005
202/639-8140
Contact this group to order a copy of its 32-page booklet "A Consumer Guide to Hospice Care," which in- *cludes a consumer checklist, information on reimbursement, and case histories, or send $4.*

Social Security Administration
Baltimore, MD 21235
For more information on Medicare benefits, including the Medicare hospice benefit, consult The Medicare Handbook *and the government*

151

pamphlet entitled "Medicare Hospice Benefits"; or else contact your nearest Social Security Administration office or call:
Toll-free: 800/772-1213

Hospice Groups

National Hospice Organization
1901 N. Moore Street
Suite 901
Arlington, VA 22209
703/243-5900
For referrals to hospices in your area, call: 800/658-8898
National organization for hospice care and for hospice providers.

Hospice Association of America
519 C Street NE
Washington, DC 20002
202/546-4759
A subsidiary of the National Association for Home Care.

Hospice Education Institute
Five Essex Square
P.O. Box 713
Essex, CT 06426
203/767-1620
"Hospice Link" toll-free hotline:
800/331-1620
Referrals to a regularly updated directory of hospice and palliative care programs nationwide, plus general information on hospice care and information on bereavement issues and services.

Academy of Hospice Physicians
500 9th Street N
Suite 200
St. Petersburg, FL 33075
813/823-8899
Offers referrals to hospice physicians nationwide.

International Hospice Institute
15801 Providence Drive
Suite 10-C
Southfield, MI 48075
313/559-4733
Provides information on hospice care.

National Institute for Jewish Hospice
8723 Alden Drive
Suite 652
Los Angeles, CA 90048
Toll-free: 800/446-4448 (nationally except California)
213/HOSPICE (467-7423)
(in California)

Children with Life-threatening Illnesses

Children's Hospice International
901 N. Washington Street
Alexandria, VA 22314
703/684-0330
Toll-free: 800/24-CHILD
(242-4453)
Information on children's hospice care for the general public, referrals to

local hospice programs or other health professionals, and printed materials.

The Candlelighters Childhood
Cancer Foundation
7910 Woodmont Avenue
Suite 460
Bethesda, MD 20814
301/657-8401
Toll-free: 800/366-2223
For families of children or adolescents with cancer and survivors of childhood cancer; provides education, peer support, an information clearinghouse, referrals to local contacts, publications, and advocacy.

The Compassionate Friends
P.O. Box 3696
Oak Brook, IL 60522
708/990-0010
Self-help organization for families that have lost a child.

Cancer Information

National Cancer Institute
Cancer Information Services
Toll-free: 800/4-CANCER
(422-6237)
National directory of information on cancer, referral to local support groups and other resources; also has information on pain management.

American Cancer Society
1599 Clifton Road NE
Atlanta, GA 30329

Toll-free: 800/ACS-2345
(227-2345)
Cancer response system for the public, patients, and families; referrals to local ACS offices.

AIDS Information

Federal Centers for Disease
Control
National AIDS Hotline
1600 Clifton Road N.E.
Atlanta, GA 30333
Toll-free: 800/342-2437
En Espanol: 800/344-7432
Hearing impaired, TTY, TTD:
800/243-7889
Primary government information source on AIDS.

People with AIDS Coalition
31 W. 26th Street
New York, NY 10010
212/532-0568
Toll-free: 800/828-3280
Referral service; information on AIDS.

National Association of People
with AIDS
1413 K Street NW
Tenth Floor
Washington, DC 20005
202/898-0414
Information, referrals, and advocacy.

Mothers of AIDS Patients
P.O. Box 1763
Lomita, CA 90717

310/542-3019
For families and concerned others, not just mothers; information, referrals, networking, and support groups.

Other Life-threatening Illnesses

Amyotrophic Lateral Sclerosis (ALS) Association
21021 Ventura Boulevard
Suite 321
Woodland Hills, CA 91364
818/340-7500
The only national organization dedicated solely to the fight against ALS (Lou Gehrig's disease); provides local referrals for counseling, training, and support.

Alzheimer's Association
919 N. Michigan Avenue
Suite 100
Chicago, IL 60611
312/335-8700
Toll free: 800/272-3900
Referrals to 217 local chapters nationwide.

Pain Management

National Chronic Pain Outreach Association
7979 Old Georgetown Road
Suite 100
Bethesda, MD 20814
301/652-4948

Information clearinghouse about chronic pain and its management; publications; and referrals to pain management specialists, pain clinics, and pain support groups.

American Chronic Pain Association
P.O. Box 850
Rocklin, CA 95677
916/632-0922
Offers a support system for those suffering chronic pain, guidelines for selecting a pain management unit, and referrals to 600 chapters internationally.

Pain Management Information Center
301 Harris B. Dates Drive
Ithaca, NY 14850
Toll-free: 800/322-PMIC (322-7642)
Mostly intended for health professionals, but will share information and written materials with the public; for cancer pain only — not other types of pain.

Wisconsin Cancer Pain Initiative
1300 University Avenue
Room 3675
Madison, WI 53706
608/262-0978
Limited staffing, not a consulting service, but can provide information, printed materials, and assistance in establishing cancer pain initiatives in other states.

Funeral Planning

National Funeral Directors
Association
11121 W. Oklahoma Avenue
Milwaukee, WI 53227
414/541-2500
Information on hospice and on funeral preplanning, prearranging, and cremation options.

Continental Association of
Funeral and Memorial Societies
6900 Lost Lake Road
Egg Harbor, WI 54209
414/868-3136
Toll-free: 800/458-5563
Information for arranging simple, inexpensive funerals.

Living Wills

Choice in Dying
200 Varick Street
New York, NY 10014
212/366-5540
Formerly called Concern for

Dying/Society for the Right to Die; provides information on living wills and other advance directives in every state, plus sample living wills.

Grief Resources

Widowed Persons' Service
American Association of Retired
Persons
601 E Street NW
Washington, DC 20049
202/434-2260
Referrals to local grief support services, publications, and audiovisual resources; for all widowed persons, not just AARP members or the elderly.

THEOS Foundation, Inc.—They
Help Each Other Spiritually
1301 Clark Building
717 Liberty Avenue
Pittsburgh, PA 15222
412/471-7779
For widows and widowers; information and referral to local chapters.

NOTES ON THE TEXT
AND SUGGESTIONS
FOR FURTHER
READING

Introduction

Sandol Stoddard's quote comes from *The Hospice Movement: A Better Way of Caring for the Dying* (New York: Stein & Day, 1978), which is also the source for the epigraph by Cicely Saunders at the beginning of this book. Stoddard's book introduced hospice care to the American public back in the movement's early days, and it remains the clearest and most evocative account of the historical and philosophical underpinnings of the modern hospice movement. Many other books about hospice have been published since Stoddard's, but most are targeted at health care policy makers, hospice administrators, hospice professionals, or others interested in establishing new hospice programs. One other book on hospice that might be of interest to a motivated lay reader is *The Hospice Alternative: A New Context for Death and Dying*, by

Anne Munley (New York: Basic Books, 1983), based on the six months Munley spent as a participant/observer at an unnamed U.S. hospice. A helpful summary of the hospice movement's historical antecedents and principles is *Nursing Care of the Terminally Ill*, edited by Madelon O'Rawe Amenta and Nancy L. Bohnet (Boston: Little, Brown and Company, 1986), and Larry R. Churchill's "The Ethics of Hospice Care," in *The Hospice: Development and Administration*, edited by Glen W. Davidson (Washington, D.C.: Hemisphere Publications, second edition, 1985), also discusses the values embedded in the hospice concept. *On Death and Dying*, by Elisabeth Kubler-Ross (New York: Macmillan, 1969), based on her interviews with dying patients, is the landmark study of the modern phenomenon of dying in America, including the treatment of dying patients in hospitals.

Chapter One: What Is Hospice Care?

This chapter summarizes key concepts from my interviews with hospice professionals in Kentucky and Wisconsin in April and May of 1991. Definitions and descriptions of hospice care can also be found in "The Basics of Hospice Care," a brochure published by the National Hospice Organization (NHO), Arlington, Virginia, and "Standards for a Hospice Program of Care" (NHO, 1987).

Chapter Two: For Whom Is Hospice Intended?

The cancer statistics come from "Cancer Facts and Figures: 1991," a booklet published by the American Cancer Society, Atlanta, Georgia. Hospice statistics are from the 1990 National Hospice Census, conducted by the National Hospice Organization, and from *NHO Newsline*, December

15, 1991. The six requirements for enrollment in hospice are composites drawn from a number of individual hospices' brochures, policies, and consent forms. Requirement four, the need for a safe setting for care, is my own phrasing of various hospice admission policies sharing this basic goal, most often stated as a requirement for the presence of a family caregiver and a safe home. A good summary of the issues around telling dying patients the truth about their diagnosis is "Therapeutic Uses of Truth," by Michael A. Simpson, in *The Dying Patient: The Medical Management of Incurable and Terminal Illness*, edited by Eric Wilkes (Ridgewood, New Jersey: George A. Bogden & Sons, 1982). Sources on the Patient Self-Determination Act include *The PSDA Handbook: Hospice Edition* (compiled and published by the California Consortium on Patient Self-Determination, Los Angeles, California, September, 1991), and "Preserving Patient Self-Determination," by Beresford, in *California Hospice Report*, Winter 1991/92.

Chapter Three: The Services Provided by a Hospice

This chapter's description of hospice services and teamwork is drawn from the interviews and from hospice brochures and booklets such as "Hospice: A Manual for Patients and Families," published by Kaiser Permanente Hospice, Walnut Creek, California; and "Hospice: A Special Kind of Caring: Handbook for Families Facing a Terminal Illness," by Pat Herrington and Jim Ewens, published by Milwaukee Hospice Home Care. Hospice services under Medicare are also summarized in "Medicare Hospice Benefits," a brochure published by the U.S. Department of Health and Human Services. The author has observed numerous hospice team meetings at Visiting Nurses and Hospice of San Francisco over the years. *Nursing Care of the Terminally Ill*, by Amenta and Bohnet, outlines the hospice nurse's skilled assessment process and responsibilities in symptom management. Stephen Connor's comment on personal care aides is from "The Hospice Home Health Aide: Hired Help, or Team Player?" by Beresford, in *Hospice Magazine*, Fall 1990. Janet Clyde's comment on volunteers is from "What Motivates Hospice Volunteers?" by Beresford, in *NHO Hospice News*, November/December, 1988.

Chapter Four: Additional Hospice Services

A compilation of the features characterizing hospice in-patient units is in "Home and Nature Links Highlight Hospices," by Deborah Allen Carey, in *Hospitals* magazine, February 16, 1984. Limitations on inpatient hospice care are discussed in "Freestanding In-Patient Hospices," by Beresford, *California Hospice Report*, Fall 1991. The author is a patient care volunteer at Coming Home Hospice, a residential hospice facility operated by Visiting Nurses and Hospice of San Francisco. *Developing AIDS Residential Settings: A Manual*, by Bill Haskell, Norma Satten, Pat Franks, and Jeannee Parker Martin (published by Visiting Nurses and Hospice of San Francisco in 1988) also outlines the continuum of inpatient and residential care settings for terminally ill patients. The discussion of nursing home/hospice collaborations is drawn in part from "Adding Value in Nursing Home Contracting," by Beresford, in *California Hospice Report*, Spring 1992.

The basic goals of hospice bereavement programs and the list of bereavement services are composites drawn from the interviews; from hospice brochures and booklets such as "After the Loss" (published by Visiting Nurses and Hospice of San Francisco); and from *Bridging the Bereavement Gap,* by Donna O'Toole (Lapeer, Michigan: The Bereavement Project, Lapeer Area Hospice, 1985). *Bereavement: Reactions, Consequences, and Care,* by Marian Osterweis, Fredric Soloman and Morris Green, (Washington, D.C.: National Academy Press, 1984) is a thorough examination of contemporary knowledge on grief, as well as research on grief services, including hospice. *Grief Counseling and Grief Therapy: A Handbook for the Mental Health Practitioner,* by J. William Worden (New York: Springer Publishing Co., 1982), describes the basic emotional tasks which need to be completed by a bereaved person. A recent article by Camille Wortman and Roxane Silver, "The Myths of Coping with Loss," in *Journal of Consulting and Clinical Psychology* (Volume 57, Number 3, 1989), reviews recent grief research to underscore the fact that there is no one "right" or "normal" pattern for grief, either in terms of intensity or duration of the individual's grief response.

✏ *Chapter Five: The Referral Process*

Especially helpful insights on the meaning of the hospice decision, and the process of the hospice referral, for both this chapter and the Afterword, came from conversations with William Carter, admissions coordinator for Lourdes Hospice in Paducah, Kentucky; Marsha Sherman, oncology social worker at Saint Joseph Hospital in Lexington, Kentucky; and Joseph Ousley, M.D., medical director for St. Joseph's Medical Center Hospice in Marshfield, Wisconsin. The author was also privileged to accompany Carter and Judy Sandler, clinical coordinator for Hospice of the Bluegrass in Lexington, on hospice intake visits to newly referred patients. The physician's role in hospice referrals is documented in *The Hospice Decision: Multiple Determinants,* final report published June 30, 1986, by

Gordon Bonham, David Gochman, Linda Burgess, and A. M.
Frean of the University of Louisville Urban Studies Center.

☙ Chapter Six: Hospice Providers, Coverage, and Access Issues

The author's formulation of the models of hospice programs
is based on *Hospice Creative Contracting and Case Management
of the Terminally Ill: Final Public Report and Manual* (published
in 1987 by Hospice of San Joaquin, Stockton, California).
Issues of certification, accreditation, and licensure for hos-
pice are summarized in "Hospice Movement Loses Its
Accreditation Program," by Beresford, in NHO *Hospice News*,
May/June 1990. The account of the passage of the Medicare
hospice benefit is drawn from "NHO: History of the National
Hospice Organization, 1978–1988," a booklet published in
1989 by the National Hospice Organization, Arlington,
Virginia, and from conversations with Donald Gaetz, Vice
Chairman, VITAS Innovative Hospice Services, Miami,
Florida, and others involved in its passage. Information on
private insurance benefits for hospice care comes from
"Growing Pains for Hospices," by Beresford, in *Business &
Health*, September 1990, from a patient information brochure
and other published materials of Milwaukee Hospice Home
Care, and from conversations with that agency's director,
James Ewens. Questions that consumers can ask their hospice
were drawn in part from *Dying at Home: A Family Guide for
Caregiving*, by Andrea Sankar (Baltimore: The Johns Hopkins
University Press, 1991), and "A Consumer Guide to Hospice
Care," a booklet published by the National Consumers
League, Washington, D.C. Barriers to hospice in rural areas
are described in "Rural Hospice Care: Problems and
Solutions," by Beresford, in *California Hospice Report*, Winter

1990. The discussion of barriers for minorities is based on "How Much Outreach to Minorities is Enough?" by Beresford, in *NHO Hospice News*, February 1990, and on conversations with Bernice Catherine Harper, chair of NHO's Task Force on Access to Hospice Care by Minorities; Carolyn Fitzpatrick-Cassin, director, Hospice of Southeastern Michigan, Southfield; and Audrey Gordon, assistant professor, University of Illinois at Chicago School of Public Health. Gordon's research is contained in *Results of a National Study of Hospice and Minorities* (unpublished).

🕸 *Chapter Seven: Pain and Physical Realities*

In-depth discussions of the realities of caring for a dying loved one at home, and of the stresses of the caregiver's role, can be found in two recent books, Sankar's *Dying at Home: A Family Guide for Caregiving*, and *Coming Home: A Guide to Dying at Home with Dignity*, by Deborah Duda (New York: Aurora Press, 1987). The hospice approach to pain management is well summarized in "The Physical Control of Pain," by Derek Doyle, in *Palliative Care: The Management of Far-Advanced Illness*, edited by Doyle (Philadelphia: Charles Press, 1984), which is quoted several times in this chapter. Balfour Mount's foreword to Doyle's book is the source for Mount's epigraph. Eric J. Cassell's landmark article "The Nature of Suffering and the Goals of Medicine," in *New England Journal of Medicine* (March 18, 1982), was recently expanded into a book with the same title (New York: Oxford University Press, 1991). For Derek Humphry's viewpoint, see his *Final Exit: The Practicalities of Self-Deliverance and Assisted Suicide* (Eugene, Oregon: The Hemlock Society, 1991). Other valuable sources on the relief of pain and other physical symptoms of terminal illness include: *Notes on Symptom*

Control in Hospice and Palliative Care, by Peter Kaye (Essex, Connecticut: Hospice Education Institute, 1990); *R. V. H. Manual on Palliative/Hospice Care: A Resource Book,* edited by Ina Ajamian and Balfour Mount (New York: Arno Press, 1980); *Hospice: Complete Care for the Terminally Ill,* by Jack M. Zimmerman (Baltimore: Urban & Schwarzenberg, 1986); and *Care of the Dying,* by Richard Lamerton (Westport, Connecticut: Technomic Publication Company, 1973).

Chapter Eight: Legal Issues

See notes for Chapter 2, above, on the PSDA; the Sankar and Duda books on caregiving; and "Why I Don't Have a Living Will," by Joanne Lynn, *Law, Medicine & Health Care,* Spring/Summer, 1991.

Chapter Nine: The Place for Hope in Hospice

Avery Weisman's epigraph is from *On Dying and Denying: A Psychiatric Study of Terminality* (New York: Behavioral Publications, 1972). Stephen Connor's comments are from a 1987 interview with the author, and from "Denial, Acceptance and Other Myths," in *Death, Dying and Bereavement: Lessons for the Living,* edited by I. Corless, B. Germino, and M. Pittman-Lindeman (Boston: Jones & Bartlett, in press). William and Susan Buchholz gave a presentation on "Hope, False Hope and Denial" at the National Hospice Organization's 13th Annual Meeting in Seattle, Washington, November, 1991.

Chapter Ten: Issues in the Future of Hospice

Information on the home infusion therapy industry is from "The Home IV Infusion Therapy Market," in *Spectrum: Health*

Care Delivery (Burlington, Massachusetts: Decision Re-
sources, June 26, 1990). Michael Levy's comment is from
"Decision-Making Dilemmas Over High-Tech Treatment," by
Beresford, *NHO Hospice News*, November, 1990. Current information on AIDS and hospice care comes from a special is-
sue devoted to this subject in *The Hospice Journal*, Volume 7,
Numbers 1 and 2, 1991, edited by Madalon O'Rawe Amenta.
Claire Tehan's comments and figures come from "The Cost of
Caring for Patients with HIV Infection in Hospice," in that
special issue. The author has interviewed staff at Visiting
Nurses and Hospice of San Francisco numerous times about
their agency's services for people with AIDS — dating back to
1984, when he was the agency's public relations coordinator.
VNHSF executive director Jeannee Parker Martin and team
leaders Mark Donnell and Kathleen Cummings were also interviewed in February 1992. Another source is *AIDS Home
Care and Hospice Manual*, by Anne Hughes, Jeannee Parker
Martin, and Pat Franks (published by VNHSF in 1987).
Children's Hospice International in Alexandria, Virginia, and
its director, Ann Armstrong Dailey, are sources for the section
on hospice and children.